Foundations in Nursing and Health Care

Communication in Clinical Settings

Paul Crawford, Brian Brown and Paul Bonham

Series Editor: Lynne Wigens

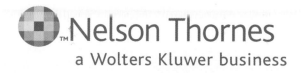

Nelson Thornes
a Wolters Kluwer business

Published in 2006 by:
Nelson Thornes Ltd
Delta Place
27 Bath Road
CHELTENHAM
GL53 7TH
United Kingdom

06 07 08 09 10 / 10 9 8 7 6 5 4 3 2 1

A catalogue record for this book is available from the British Library

ISBN-10: 0 7487 9716 5
ISBN-13: 978 0 7487 9716 5

Illustrations by Clinton Banbury and Eugene Osborne
Page make-up by Florence Production Ltd

Printed and bound in Slovenia by Korotan-Ljubljana

For Owen Robert
With love

Acknowledgements

We would like to thank all our academic colleagues, especially members of the Health Language Research Group at the University of Nottingham. Thank you also to Lisa Fraley, our series editor Lynne Wigens and the reviewers who gave us the chance to write this book. Finally we thank the wider community of scholars and writers who have contributed to knowledge about communication in health care.

Thanks to the British Deaf Association for permission to use the finger spelling alphabet.

Every effort has been made to contact copyright holders and the publishers apologise to anyone whose rights have been overlooked and will be happy to rectify any errors or omissions.

Contents

Preface

In this book we suggest the need for a change in how we communicate in health care practice and introduce a new model: Brief, Ordinary and Effective (BOE). This model is an attempt to promote an ongoing and consistent level of warm, positive communication in clinical settings and challenges the all-too-familiar claim that communicating with patients takes far too much time. This sense of communication as a 'time-greedy' activity owes much to the domination of counselling models more suited to mental health contexts rather than busy general clinical settings. The BOE model also promotes the value of engaging in ordinary ways with people and attending to what users of health services and research evidence suggest are the most effective kinds of interaction. The core BOE skills listed in the final chapter can be used as a useful checklist to aid regular reflection and monitoring of communication work in health settings. The BOE model informed the Department of Health's recent guidelines on best practice in mental health nursing (Department of Health 2006) and several NHS trusts are considering adapting this model that has been in responce to Essence of Care initiatives. It is a model that has been designed to shape or direct communication in all clinical settings, not sinply mental health care.

The skills involved in communicating with others are complex and this book is not meant to be comprehensive. We hope it provides a helpful and interesting introduction to communicating in clinical settings and gets you thinking about the key issues. We have tried to offer some of the main ingredients for successful interpersonal working with patients, their relatives and health professionals.

We consider that many interpersonal skills are already available to us as we develop and grow into adulthood, and experience all kinds of interactions both inside and outside health settings, but that reflection on how we communicate and the language we use can help us to refine and advance the work we do with patients. Of course, some aspects of communicating, for example in dealing with very challenging situations, may require further specialist training.

This book draws upon and builds from a number of our earlier publications in the field of health communication, not least: Crawford *et al.* (1998) *Communicating Care: The Language of Nursing* (Stanley Thornes); Crawford, R., Brown, B. and Crawford, P. (2004) *Storytelling in Therapy* (Nelson Thornes); Bonham, P (2004) *Communicating as a Mental Health Carer* (Nelson Thornes); Crawford, P. and Brown, B. (2004) 'Communication' in: Mallik, M, Hall, C. and Howard, D. (eds) *Nursing Knowledge and Practice: Foundations for Decision Making*. 2nd edition. Edinburgh: Balliere Tindall. It also points to and complements theoretical debates covered in: Brown, *et al.* (2006) *Evidence Based Health Communication* (Open University Press).

Paul Crawford, Nottingham
2006

References

Department of Health (2006) *Best practice competencies and capabilities for pre-registration mental health nurses in England. The Chief Nursing Officer's review of mental health nursing*. Stationary Office, London.

1 Physical, psychological and social aspects of communication

Learning outcomes

By the end of this chapter you should be able to:

- Identify theories and models of communication
- Describe the sensory organs and the interpretation of language and non-verbal signals in the brain
- Demonstrate insight into ideas about how and why human beings come to be language users
- Appreciate the positive and negative styles of communication used by nurses and other health professionals
- Identify strategies for dealing with a variety of communication difficulties
- Identify psychosocial factors affecting communication
- Appreciate interplay between culture, narratives and metaphors of health and illness

Introduction

Communication is a powerful action that can change people's lives for better or worse. For example, just think for a moment how we can make someone feel good by commenting positively on their clothing or how a child's confidence can be destroyed by a cruel nickname. Think how we can lift a person emotionally through a genuine smile, comforting touch or simply by using eye contact to let someone know that they are not invisible. The truth is that we use all kinds of **non-verbal** and **verbal** spoken or written communication in our many roles in professional life. For example, we use various facial expressions and **gestures** and adopt particular **postures**. We speak or listen to others, write or read words, create or view images and symbols. All this activity – and it is an activity – is communication. We are always communicating – even in our silence. We can't help it! It is what makes us fully human. But this fundamental or key aspect of being human requires careful attention and consideration. Communication can help us achieve so many things but it can also damage other people. If we take our caring work seriously then we must continue to respect the power of communication to change lives and harness the skills to communicate more effectively.

Whatever our clinical focus – adult, mental health, learning disabilities, child – very different results can emerge from the process of caring for others depending on how communication is carried out. How we and others communicate will have a great impact on the quality of care. It is worth reminding ourselves that despite our pride in caring work, poor communication in clinical settings is the largest source of patient dissatisfaction (Carls-Verhallen *et al.* 1999). This is disappointing and suggests that we need to invest much more in our skills and strategies for communicating if we are to retain our core tradition of caring for others – something addressed in the Department of Health's

○━╥ *Keywords*

Verbal/Non-verbal
Communication that uses or
does not use spoken or written
words

Gesture
The use of the body, such as
the hand, as an expression of
thought or feeling

Posture
The relative position of parts of
the body

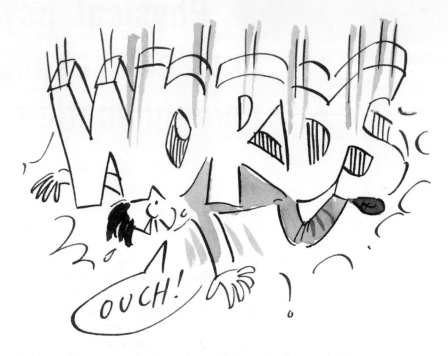

Sticks and stones may break my bones, but words will never hurt me.

11 benchmarks for best practice in communication between
patients, carers and health care personnel (Department of Health
2003) (see box below).

Essence of care – benchmarks of best practice in communication

1. All health care personnel demonstrate effective interpersonal skills when
   communicating with patients and or carers
2. Communication takes place at a time and in an environment that is acceptable
   to all parties
3. All patients' and or carers' communication needs are assessed on initial
   contact and are regularly reassessed. Additional communication support is
   negotiated and provided when a need is identified
4. Information that is accessible, acceptable, up to date and meets the needs of
   individuals is shared actively and consistently with all patients and or carers
   and widely promoted across all communities
5. Appropriate and effective methods of communication are used actively to
   promote understanding between patients and or carers and health care
   personnel
6. The principal carer is identified at all times and an assessment is made with
   them of their needs, involvement, willingness and ability to collaborate with
   practitioners in order to provide care

7. All patients and/or carers are continuously supported and fully enabled to perform their role safely

8. All care providers communicate fully and effectively with each other to ensure that patients and/or carers benefit from a comprehensive plan of care which is regularly updated and evaluated

9. All patients and/or carers are enabled to communicate their individual needs and preferences at all times

10. Effective communication ensures and demonstrates that the patients' and/or carers' expert contribution to patient care is valued, recorded and informs both patient care and health care personnel education

11. All the patients' and/or carers' information, support and training needs are jointly identified, agreed, met and regularly reviewed

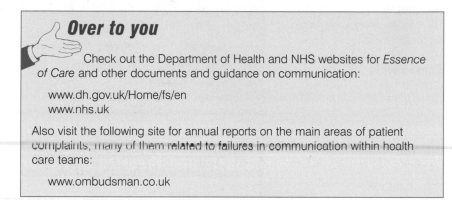

Over to you

Check out the Department of Health and NHS websites for *Essence of Care* and other documents and guidance on communication:

www.dh.gov.uk/Home/fs/en
www.nhs.uk

Also visit the following site for annual reports on the main areas of patient complaints, many of them related to failures in communication within health care teams:

www.ombudsman.co.uk

Nursing is an interpersonal process in which we aim to identify and use common meanings in our communication with others; work in a collaborative way; and interpret the health needs of others. As nurses, the ways in which we communicate can have profound effects on the people around us. Our communication shapes and transforms clinical settings, establishes who we are, and who others are in relation to us. Let us begin by examining the major trends and topics in the study of communication and explore the implications for nursing practice.

Reflective activity

List the kinds of communication you have taken part in during the last week – e.g. speaking, listening, writing, reading, non-verbal, graphical (drawing), symbolic. What did your communication do? How would you measure success or failure in your communication with others?

Key points ~~Top tips~~

- Communication is a powerful action that can change people's lives for better or worse
- We use all kinds of non-verbal and verbal/spoken or written communication in our many roles in professional life
- Poor communication in clinical settings is the largest source of patient dissatisfaction
- Our communication shapes and transforms clinical settings, establishes who we are, and who others are in relation to us

O─┱ Keywords

Autonomy
The right to self-government or personal freedom

Empowering
Giving power to

~~Key points~~ Top tips

Avoid being 'powerful' or authoritarian in communicating with patients and clients by:
- Respecting their **autonomy** and view of the world
- Using dignified, ordinary or everyday language
- **Empowering** them through information giving and involvement in decision-making

Models and theories of communication

Communication is something we do in our internal world of thoughts and in the external world by speaking, writing, gestures, drawing, making images and symbols or receiving messages from others.

The basis of communication is fairly simple and can be summarised in the following model: sender, message and receiver. For example, a nurse (sender) says 'Good morning' (message) to a patient who hears the greeting (receiver). But the mechanics of how this takes place are much more complex and there are various models or frameworks for understanding such activity.

The transmission and transaction models

O─┱ Keywords

Transmission
A one way transfer of information

One-way flow

The one-way **transmission** model originated by Shannon and Weaver (1949), views communication as a transfer of meaning from one person to another as if down a pipe or wire. This model is now considered as rather limited. It does not capture the interactive aspect of communication.

⊙—🔑 Keywords

Transaction(al)

Two-way communication or dialogue

Two way flow

A better model of communication is offered in what is called a two-way or **transactional** model of communication (Ratzan *et al.* 1996). This involves dialogue between sender and receiver where shared meaning and mutual understanding grows. Words and their meaning are not simply deposited like a box of goods with the receiver. Instead we have a kind of 'ping-pong' exchange between people that is subject to their different beliefs, values, assumptions and prejudices. In this two-way activity we work hard to interpret each other or decode what the other person means by their words.

Communication: context and intention

⊙—🔑 Keywords

Context

Situations, activities or events surrounding communication

Another way of making sense of communication is to consider the context and purpose for sender and message (Jakobson 1960). Here we are concerned with how the **context** or circumstances in which we communicate determines the meaning of any message. Rather like wearing different clothing, we adopt a variety of styles of communicating to suit a range of contexts and situations and for any number of purposes. In so doing, we are usually versatile, often tailoring our communication to suit the situation. For example, we are likely to communicate rather differently at a party, or with an intimate partner, than at a job interview or during a staff meeting on a ward.

Language as an activity – speech acts

⊙—🔑 Keywords

Speech act

Use of language for a particular purpose or to achieve something in particular

Whenever we communicate, we act. We do things with our words and expressions. For example, our speech will often have a purpose such as praising, warning, promising, or apologising, etc. Searle (1979) calls these **speech acts**. In addition, it is through our communication with others that we establish our persona or identity – we construct who we are. Sumner (2001) argues that when these communicative actions in nursing are successful, they lead to a sense of fulfilment and validation for client and carer.

Reflective activity

Think about a recent communication with someone. What were you trying to achieve in the interaction? What were you trying to get the other person/people to do? What were they trying to get you to do?

Write a brief analysis of an episode of communication you had with a patient and/or a colleague. Try to identify what actions were performed in your speech – e.g. advising, informing, counselling, warning, etc.

Language builds our realities – social construction

Another way of looking at our communication is in terms of building or constructing reality in clinical settings. As Potter (1996) demonstrates, versions of reality can be created through the language we use. The kind of talk and other forms of communication in any clinical setting will build a particular environment or reality for ourselves and those we care for. This might be a supportive, warm 'reality', or it may be cold and rejecting. It might be dominated by the language of professionals or it may allow the patient or client to have a voice. How people communicate and what they choose to communicate about will, in other words, create a particular form of reality. Another way of thinking about this is to consider communication in the same way as a physical intervention, or as real as the equipment or architecture of a clinical setting. As with décor, our communication can be designed and altered to achieve particular effects. We build communicative landscapes for our patients and clients.

This **social construction** model of communication may sound abstract, but it is a useful way to think about the process of interaction in clinical settings. For example, Bricher (1999, p. 453) describes how trust can be constructed between nurses and sick children. As one of her respondents said:

'I show them a photo of my dog and they realise . . . that you've got a backyard and a dog too, like [you are] not just this person that sticks suppositories up.' The communicative landscape on offer here is one that promotes trust and allows the treatment to be undertaken with a minimum of distress, and even when a distressing procedure is undertaken, the relationship can be re-established quickly.

Keywords

Social construction
The way that social reality is organised and designed by humans according to particular viewpoints, norms or rules

Reflective activity

Think about the different communicative landscapes that you have come across in everyday settings. It might be a party, a shopping trip, a visit to a church, seeing a bank manager or going to a sports event. How is this 'communicative landscape' designed or built? Does it promote or inhibit particular actions? How does it do this? What kinds of identity or persona do you adopt in each setting?

Now think about a clinical setting you have experienced during or before your training. How is the 'communicative landscape' of the clinical area designed or built? Does it promote or inhibit particular actions? How does it do this? What kinds of identity or persona do you adopt in each setting? Finally, what kinds of identity or persona do patients or clients adopt?

Thus, we have seen so far a variety of theories related to communication, and sketched out a number of things that language may do in health care. But how do we become technically competent as communicators in the first place?

Key points ~~Top tips~~

- Communication can be internal (our thoughts) and external (interacting with others)
- The basic model of communication is that of a sender, message and receiver
- Communication can be viewed as one-way (transmission) or two-way (transaction)
- Context and purpose are key factors in communication
- Communication and the language we use can be thought of as activity or action (as speech acts)
- Language builds or constructs social and clinical realities
- Communication in clinical settings establishes our professional identity and that of patients and clients

~~Key points~~ **Top tips**

Always approach communication as:
- an opportunity to share meanings
- an action with consequences
- potentially life-transforming

The biological bases of communication

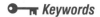 *Keywords*

Medium
The means through which we communicate or represent things

Communication has its base in human anatomy and physiology. In speech, the mouth, nose, pharynx, epiglottis, trachea and lungs combine to produce particular kinds of sound that make up the **medium** for conveying messages to others. With our complex anatomy, not least our ears, eyes, and particular muscles, we are enabled to do such things as type on a keyboard, write, or produce and receive a vast range of verbal and non-verbal messages – all facilitated by a variety of neurological processes. Let us examine those in a little more detail, beginning with a summary of mechanisms of speech.

Mechanisms of speech

We speak by pushing air out of our lungs, through the trachea (or 'windpipe') into the larynx ('Adam's apple'), where vocal cords take up one of two positions. When they are drawn together like a stiff pair of curtains, the air from our lungs has to be forced through and this causes a vibration. If you place a finger on the top of the larynx and produce 'voiced' sounds like [z] you will experience this sensation. When the vocal cords are left apart like loose curtains, air moves through to make 'voiceless' sounds such as [s] or [f], where there is no vibration.

The air passing through the larynx moves into the mouth and/or nose. Consonant sounds, for example [m] in *marriage* or [p] in *pillow*, are formed by changing the shape of the oral cavity, notably with the tongue. Try out the following articulations and determine which sounds are 'voiced' or 'voiceless':

Alveolars – Sounds like [t] in *top* or [n] in *nut* are made with the tip of the tongue on the alveolar ridge at the front of the hard palate.

Alveo-palatals – Sounds like [ch] in *cheeky* and [sh] in *shoot* are made by placing the tongue at the front of the palate.

Bilabials – Sounds like [b] in *batter* or [p] in *pudding* are made by using both upper and lower lips.

Dentals – Sounds like [th] in *thank* or *path* are made by placing the tip of the tongue behind the upper front teeth.

Glotals – Sounds like [h] in *home* or *who* are made when the space between the vocal cords or glottis is open but the sound is not shaped or manipulated by the mouth.

Labiodentals – Sounds like [f] in *fetch* and [v] in *vanish* are made with the upper teeth and lower lip.

Velars – Sounds like as [k] in *cool* or *keep* and [g] in *game* are made by pressing the back of the tongue against the velum (soft palate) at the back of the mouth. The sound [ng] in *tongue* or *sang* is formed by lowering the soft palate to let air through the nasal cavity.

Of course, these are just the positions and shapes taken in the mouth to produce sounds, but this manipulation is done in particular ways. Thus there are:

Affricates: when sounds like [ch] in *chip* are made by the friction of obstructing the release of air that has been briefly stopped.

Approximants: when sounds like [w] in *when* or [y] in *yes* are made with the tongue moving forward.

Glottal stops: when the glottis is briefly closed and released as when people speaking Cockney say *butter* or *matter* without pronouncing the 'tt' part in the middle.

Nasals: when sounds like [m], [n] or [ng] as in *snoring* are made when air is directed out through the nose.

Stops: when sounds such as [p], [b], [d], [t], [k] or [g] are produced by briefly stopping the passage of air in the mouth cavity and letting it go.

Many of the sounds produced in this way form words, but a significant proportion form what have been termed 'guggles' – the expressions of surprise, support, 'um hmm', 'ah ha' and so forth, which form part of a **paralanguage** and may be used to support and encourage a speaker or to indicate that a person wishes to interrupt. Also, they may be important in conveying emotion.

Once the sounds have been made, of course, they must be perceived for communication to take place. Sounds waves enter the ear and are converted into nervous impulses and enter the brain via the cochlear nerve. The basic anatomy of the ear is shown in Fig. 1.2 on p. 10.

Sound waves enter via the pinna and outer ear canal and vibrate the eardrum or tympanum. This transmits vibration via the bones of the ear (the hammer, anvil and stirrup) to the cochlea which is rich in nerve endings. The cochlea is able to detect the minute deformations in the tissues caused by the vibrations and turn them into nerve impulses. These impulses then pass along the auditory nerve to the midbrain and then to the auditory cortex of the temporal lobes. Whereas the processing of sound into meaningful units of communication is not well understood, it may be that

⊶ Keywords

Paralanguage
Conveying meaning through tone, pitch or accent

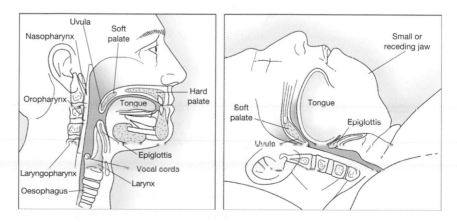

Figure 1.1 *Normal anatomy of the head and neck.*

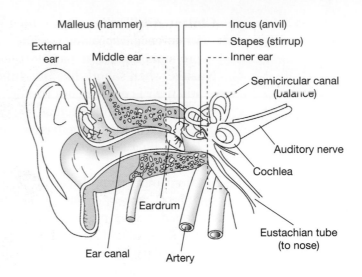

Figure 1.2 *Anatomy of the ear.*

different brain cells or groups of cells specialise in the recognition of certain kinds of sounds.

Communication and impairment

If the sensory processes themselves are impaired, this can lead to difficulties with communication. We need to consider how we can help people with sensory impairments communicate in health care settings.

There are a variety of techniques which can be used to compensate for impairments. For example, deaf people can use a number of strategies in communicating: speech, gestures, formal sign language (see Fig 1.3 on p. 11), finger-spelling, writing, reading, lip-reading and using hearing aids. Cochlear implants are an increasingly popular treatment. These involve the implantation of a device with a microphone and electrodes which stimulate the cochlear nerves directly and can provide some measure of hearing.

Over to you

For further information on hearing aid services, go to: www.mhas.info/

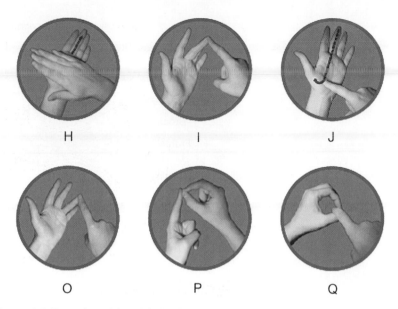

Figure 1.3 *Examples of the alphabet in sign language.*

There are a variety of aids to help visually impaired people communicate. These include: glasses, Braile, large print, books and magazines on tape, dark lined writing paper, or even a grooved writing board, through to electronic aids such as label readers or voice recognition phone diallers.

One critical aspect of non-verbal communication is the interpretation of facial expressions of emotion, and children with learning difficulties have been found to be less accurate than non-disabled children in making such interpretations. As Bandura (1986) has pointed out, the ability to read the signs of emotions in social interaction has important adaptive value in guiding actions toward others. Presumably, deficits in this area play a significant role in the social difficulties experienced by children with learning disabilities (Dimitrovsky *et al.* 1998).

Sometimes people's predispositions or inclinations may make them less likely to interpret **cues** in a particular way. For example, those who are apt to be cynical or hostile are likely to wrongly attribute happiness (Larkin *et al.* 2002). Research has also revealed gender differences in the accuracy of decoding facial expressions of emotion, with males being less accurate than females (Pell 2002).

The brain and message interpretation

The **Broca's area** in the human brain is involved in the production of speech and the **Wernicke's area** in understanding

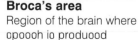
Keywords

Cues
Signals

Broca's area
Region of the brain where speech is produced

Wernicke's area
Region of the brain where speech is comprehended

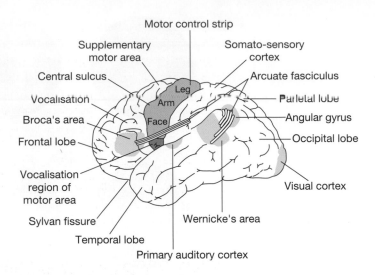

Figure 1.4 *Language areas in the brain.*

the significance of content words in speech (see Fig. 1.4). These two areas are linked by a 'motorway' of nerve fibres called the *articulate fasciculus*. Both areas have been studied closely, not least in relation to various forms of brain damage and resultant difficulties in language reception and production. Damage to Broca's area is related to difficulty in producing speech, while damage to Wernicke's area is related to speech comprehension difficulties. In addition, a part of the motor cortex, close to Broca's area, controls the muscles that articulate the face, tongue and larynx, which are key to language production, and when damaged also affect communication.

If a patient was to hear the word 'hello' and repeat it, this suggests a simple transmission of the word being heard and understood in Wernicke's area, which transfers a signal via the *articulate fasciculus* to Broca's area, where production of the word is set up with a signal being sent to the motor cortex to put it out in a physical form by moving particular muscles etc. Yet there is evidence that a large number of different areas of the brain are used for the production of spoken utterances and that different areas of the brain are activated for different aspects of speech. Hence, a rich variety of anatomical and physiological mechanisms and senses lie behind human communication. Thus, in contrast to a view of language functioning in particular parts of the brain, it appears that communication involves interdependent aspects of brain function.

Key points Top tips

- Communication has its base in human anatomy and physiology
- In speech sounds are 'voiced' or 'voiceless'
- Paralanguage ('guggles') may be used to support and encourage a speaker, indicate that a person wishes to interrupt, or express emotion
- Impaired sensory processes can lead to difficulties with communication but there are techniques and technologies that can help overcome these
- Communication is facilitated by a variety of neurological processes and involves specific parts of the brain that work interdependently in interpreting or comprehending language (Wernicke's area) and in producing speech (Broca's area)

Communication difficulties

All of us experience minor communication difficulties from time to time. Take, for example, how sound production can be hampered when you have a sore throat, a mouth ulcer, after receiving local anaesthetic at the dentist or even when your mouth is very dry.

Nurses may be called upon to work with clients with more serious communication difficulties. The nature of many illnesses is such that the client's ability to communicate is impaired, for example, and most obviously, in the case of loss of consciousness. Yet even under these circumstances, there are reports of people remembering conversations around them whilst they were apparently comatose or anaesthetised, thus highlighting the importance of ensuring that communication is appropriate. Disorders of speech may also be due to problems with anatomical mechanisms for speech (*dysarthrias*). A variety of speech and language problems arise when people suffer strokes, dementia, or have learning difficulties, sensory impairments and mental health problems, all of which may impair a person's communicative abilities. In terms of strokes, for example, it is common for the sufferer's comprehension or expression of speech to be disturbed (*receptive* or *expressive dysphasia*).

Among clients who are conscious, and attempting to recover their communication abilities, a good deal of the communication therapy may well be undertaken by a speech therapist, but often nurses will be the front line carers for such clients. There are a number of reports in the literature of nurses being able to screen patients for difficulties with chewing, drinking and swallowing (Cantwell 2000; Dumble and Tuson 1998) which may require more specialist interventions and yield improvements in communication.

As well as the technical issues of identifying impairments, nurses may be key to developing new ways of dealing with people whose communication is problematic. Bradshaw (1998) described how clinic staff developed a communication programme for a man with profound hearing loss, learning disabilities and challenging behaviour. As a result of changing their communicative actions so that there was greater use of signing and gesturing that involved a fuller range of communicative functions, staff noted that the communication skills of the man significantly improved. Staff attitudes appeared to change as they then saw him as being challenged rather than as challenging.

Training the client and the client's friends, relatives and informal caregivers to enhance the communication environment can be successfully achieved. Tye-Murray and Schurm (1994) describe how communication enhancement with individuals suffering from hearing loss can involve the rest of their family and social circle, so that 'frequent communication partners' are enabled to use more effective strategies such as clearer speaking behaviours, message tailoring and verbal repair strategies. This kind of training can also include professional carers. A variety of techniques, such as diaries and logs, can be used to help identify areas of particular difficulty and suggest strategies for improvement. On the other hand, sometimes the client and their regular communication partners can become so skilled at communicating with each other that the client has great difficulty interacting with anyone else. This may present difficulties if the client needs to go into hospital and cannot be attended by their usual carers (Erber and Scherer 1999).

Reflective activity

Nurses working in Intensive Care Units have been the subject of much research into the patterns of communication that occur with their heavily sedated and ventilated patients and they are very aware of the need for appropriate communication. Review and reflect on your experiences of communicating with patients who had difficulties:

● Reflect on how much time you spent with a patient who had communication difficulties in comparison to a patient who was able to respond normally
● Reflect on what communication patterns/styles are more effective if the patient can hear but is unable to speak to you (e.g. patient following a stroke)
● If a patient has hearing difficulties review what alterations you would make to your way of communicating
● Review your current knowledge of hearing aids such as those supplied by audiologists
● Record your learning as appropriate in your portfolio

Reciprocal
Returning or sharing (feelings, experiences)

According to Sundin *et al.* (2001) this idea that communication is concerned with the **reciprocal** or mutual interactions between clients and their carers is important. Identity is established through relationships and the loss of a person's ability to communicate threatens their sense of self. Once people's communicative ability has been impaired, perhaps through a stroke, social relationships become much more difficult. In addition, there is evidence that the prioritisation of physical care on stroke units means that nurses have less time to interact with patients (see Bennett 1996; Pound *et al.* 1995, 1999), something they find frustrating (Hemsley *et al.* 2001).

Sundin *et al.*'s (2001) study of the professional carers of people who had been disabled through stroke detected a tendency to see the patients as fragile and vulnerable; at the same time it was felt to be important to support them in a way that sustained their dignity and did not make them feel even more disabled. Equally, important parts of the caring practice with these communication-impaired patients involved developing relationships, feelings of closeness and sensitivity often involving non-verbal communication. This was seen to be achievable by spending time with the patient as a companion, not necessarily just attending to the mechanics of care. Communication, in this case, was seen to be essential to the well-being of the patients but was not possible through the normal medium of speech; instead it was accomplished through the medium of presence, trust and security. This is something that Sundin and Jansson (2003) refer to as the 'silent dialogue' in the relationship between nurses and patients.

Top tips

Communicating with care means you must:

● assess for communication disabilities

● acquire and use aids/resources to meet language or communication needs

● allow sufficient time for achieving meaningful dialogue even 'silent dialogue'

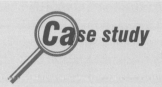

Case study

James, 68, is admitted to hospital for assessment after a fall. He appears unable or unwilling to speak and the staff on the ward struggle to make sense of his erratic and angry gestures. He resists their efforts to dress a wound to his knee and whenever they ask him questions he seems not to notice and just looks blankly ahead.

● What might be affecting the ability of James to communicate with staff?

● How will you attempt to communicate with him?

Language acquisition

Keywords
....

Syntax
The way words are put together or arranged according to grammatical rules

Grammar
The rules of a language

Innate
Something we are born with

One of the joys of being a parent is experiencing a child's development of language. It is an extraordinary process. As well as becoming competent users of a complex **syntax** determined by **grammar**, on average, English-speaking children acquire a vocabulary of about 60,000 words by the age of 18. The early stages of children's communicative learning are outlined in the table below.

During periods of peak vocabulary development a child may learn a new word every two hours! This has led some theorists (e.g. Chomsky 1976; Pinker 1994) to suggest that there are **innate** structures in the brain that enable the grammar (rules of language)

Table 1.1 Language development in children	
Child's age	**Communication development**
0–4 months	Babies start to coo and produce vowel sounds. Will make sounds back when spoken to.
6 months	Laughing. Will start to make consonant sounds like d, p and m.
6–12 months	Laughing, smiling babbling. Multi-syllable speech such as 'uh-oh', 'dadada', 'mamama'. Points to objects of interest.
12–24 months	Development of vocabulary – about 50 words by 18 months, with two-word strings such as 'hit ball' or 'see baby', or 100 by 24 months.
2–3 years	Builds sentences such as 'dada go work'. Acquires concepts like in, under or behind.
3–5 years	Development of vocabulary and syntactic ability (the grammatical arrangement of words). Phrasing requests. Sentences get longer. Working vocabulary of about 2,300 words by the age of 5 and ability to comprehend 8,000 words.

⊶ₙ Keywords

Lexicon
Collection of words, vocabulary
of a person

and **lexicon** (vocabulary) to be learned so readily. There has been much debate about whether this is the case. At the present state of knowledge, communication is far more than biology can explain. While biology may give us the mechanics as it were, it can say little about the ways that communication is employed.

Broadly speaking, messages are conveyed through our use of a rich and versatile language system. It is difficult to find a shared natural language system anywhere in the world that does not have these features. Even languages that were once believed to be 'primitive' such as sign language are now considered to be far more complex than we imagined. Indeed, gesture and facial expression are vitally important to rich communication for non-hearing and hearing cultures. Therefore, it is worth examining the issue of non-verbal communication in more detail as an awareness of these issues will enable health practitioners to become flexible and efficient communicators.

Key points

- There are key stages in a child's acquisition and development of language
- English-speaking children acquire a vocabulary of about 60,000 words by the age of 18
- There are competing views and theories as to whether language is innate or something that we learn
- Language acquisition involves the learning of grammar and development of a lexicon
- The language system is rich, versatile and complex across both hearing and non-hearing cultures

Top tips

To communicate clearly you must:
- avoid technical, abstract or difficult words
- be willing to explain or simplify complex information or procedures
- never 'speak down to' or patronise individuals
- respect the word-choice/vocabulary of others across the life-span

Psychosocial factors and communication

The kinds of communication that can take place in health settings are diverse and will involve a great variety of individuals who may have quite different viewpoints and attitudes. The way that people communicate – or, if you like, their styles of communication – will be affected by such differences and by a number of other factors, not least age, gender, social class, culture and ethnicity. Again, people will adopt different styles of speaking for different occasions. In our day-to-day lives we tend to shift between various kinds of talk, sometimes without knowing we are doing so. Consider for example, how differently we speak when socialising with friends compared to speaking with a potential employer on the telephone. When speaking with friends we tend to be informal, use slang, and may use a particular dialect and accent. When speaking to a potential employer we will tend to 'clean-up' or 'posh-up' our accent ('received pronunciation'), and use formal, official language. Similarly in health settings, we will tend to speak rather differently depending on whom we are speaking to, why we are speaking to them, where we are speaking and even when we are doing so. Our communication will be affected by the language used, rules or laws of social behaviour, the social status and power relations of participants, and the kinds of roles or life scripts that they have adopted.

Reflective activity

Observe various interactions between different health professionals and patients/clients. What do you notice? What is achieved in the communication? Who is in charge in each interaction? How do you know this? How formal or informal was the language used?

Now reflect upon your own communication with a patient/client in a health setting. Who is more powerful in the exchange?

In communication we can witness the exercise of power. This is especially the case when one of the speakers is deemed to be of higher status or is in a certain, authoritative role, such as doctor, nurse, teacher, etc. Often, professionals in health settings assert their power in talking with patients/clients. This can be associated with the ability to interrupt and take control of the 'floor' in conversation (Reid and Ng 1999). Whether through interruptions, holding a turn of conversation, or deciding what is talked about, and when a particular communication should come to an end, health professionals often position themselves in authority over patients/clients.

Refle*Reflective activity*

In what ways might health care activities, such as assessment or history-taking reveal the powerful status of the health professional?

In what ways might medical or nursing notes disadvantage patients/clients?

Do you or the patient/client close health focused conversation?

Who decides which topics are discussed in health care exchanges?

Awareness of language and communication involves an awareness of the diverse range of biological, personal and social factors which have an impact on the speech styles in use in health care. Indeed, by becoming more aware of these nurses can change the communication environment to the benefit of patients/clients and themselves.

Using language in health care

We use language in all kinds of ways in health settings and our ability to communicate will change and adapt to different contexts and demands across the lifespan. While our mission in health care tends to be one of communicating efficiently and effectively, this is not always the reality. Sadly, at times, practitioners communicate with patients and clients in limited, negative or harmful ways. The notion that language might be harmful is of particular importance in the context of health care, where the overriding aim is to promote human well-being (Crawford *et al.* 1998). It is therefore important to be aware that some styles of communication are more contentious and the role they can play in oppressing patients or clients, as well as healing them, requires careful examination.

Language as ideological and powerful

All communication takes place in particular contexts or environments and is informed and influenced by wider political and economic structures. In health care there is a wide range of professionals engaged in day-to-day communication from nurses, doctors, psychologists, occupational therapists, administrators and managers to patients, clients and their families. As such, nurses are just part of a web of communication driven or organised by powerful conceptions and ideologies of what society should be like, how it is constructed and what is important. Moreover, according to Fairclough (1989), nursing is shaped by equally powerful **ideologies** of bureaucratic 'cost-effectiveness' and 'efficiency' and nurses' training tends to promote acquiring communication or social skills

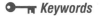 *Keywords*

Ideologies
Particular systems of ideas as ways of thinking

as a means of 'efficient people-handling' (p. 235) or what we may think of as people-processing. At times, this may mean that nurses are speaking or writing about patients and clients in a way that is not compatible with their profession's or their own value systems, but which has more to do with economics, politics and the public image of the institution for which they work.

Types of talk in health care

If we think of talk as an action – as clearly as, say, injecting someone – then we can begin to understand in more concrete terms what it is that we do with our talk and language. For what we say and how we say it can achieve very different effects. Indeed, our choice will promote or even bring into being a particular kind of reality for those we care for. For example, through our professional talk we can socialise people into rather limiting roles as 'patient', 'victim', or as someone who is in pain, simply incapable, or even as a condition (e.g. 'We have a cancer in the side room')! In other words, through our talk we can foster the varied capacities of individuals or prevent independence and autonomy. We can heal or damage with our words. We can, if you like, engage in positive or negative talk.

The positive use of talk

An example of positive talk comes from a study by Proctor *et al.* (1996) of how nurses in a Trauma Centre in a US hospital communicate with injured patients. The authors identified what they called the Comfort Talk Register, whereby different kinds of talk had specific pragmatic functions: holding on, assessing, informing and caring:

- *Holding on* was conducted through the use of phrases like 'big girl', 'you're doing great', 'count to three' that served to praise, to let the patient know they can get through, to support, to instruct or distract the patient

- *Assessing* involved 'How are you?' questions or giving the patient information such as, 'You're in the emergency room'. These involved getting information, explaining the situation or validating and confirming the patient's input

- *Informing* were statements like, It's gonna hurt' or 'We'll be inserting a catheter', that is, warning the patient or explaining procedures

- *Caring* included reassuring, empathic or caring statements like 'Relax' or 'OK sweetie' or 'It does hurt, doesn't it?'

Proctor *et al.* (1996) suggest that because these features of comfort talk are regularly used, the talk has a rhythmical, sing-song quality and is mainly used to get patients to endure the situation a little longer. The researchers highlight the importance of the style and content of communication in the commencement of courses of treatment, and indicate real benefits of using comfort talk in terms of reduced mortality rates.

Reflective activity

Observe a few clinical situations or procedures and imagine that you are watching a play or television drama:

● What is the storyline or plot for each 'drama'? Who plays the 'main role'?
● What are the similarities or differences in the way individuals act their parts?
● How do the 'dramas' end?
● How active was the patient in the way the storyline developed?
● Were any fixed or formulaic expressions used, e.g. 'What seems to be the trouble?'

The negative use of talk

An example of negative talk is the use of 'baby talk' by nurses and other carers in their interactions with elderly clients. There have been widespread complaints about this kind of controlling, institutional talk that has been observed as the use of high pitched, short utterances, interrogatives (questions) and imperatives (commands), with simple grammatical structures (de Wilde and de Ambady *et al.* 2002; Bot 1989). Perhaps surprisingly, there is some evidence to suggest that the use of this **patronising speech** style does not depend on the status of the patient as the confused are no more likely to be patronised than those who are alert and oriented. Rather, the speech style seemed to depend on the attitudes of the caregiver (Caporael *et al.* 1983).

The features of speech and non-verbal behaviour – for example high pitch, pats on the shoulder and expressions like 'that's a good girl' – are not only perceived by the elderly residents themselves as patronising, but are also seen to be unfavourable by observers (Ryan *et al.* 1994). It is important that those working with elderly people are aware of the tendency of carers to talk in these ways and that some instruction on these matters is incorporated into their education (Ryan *et al.* 1994).

⚷ Keywords

Patronising speech
Condescending talk, 'speaking down' to a person

Albert Robillard (1996), who is both a sociologist and suffers multiple disabilities, movingly describes the effects of patronising talk. He writes:

⌐⊶ *Keywords*

Interlocutor
A person who takes part in a
conversation

> The response of my **interlocutors** to my visible anger ranges from 'I did not know you could hear', 'I didn't know you could think!', 'Most of my patients are stroke victims and have trouble understanding me', to 'Oh, I am sorry, I won't do it again'. Most react to my outburst by ignoring me, leading me to see the ignoral as a further documentary reading of my symptomatology by my interlocutor. It is a toss up if my harsh reaction will change the course of interaction. Frequently those who say 'I did not know you could . . .', or 'I am sorry, I will not do it again,' go back to exclusionary practices in a few moments.
>
> (Robillard 1996, p. 19)

Much can be learned from attempting to make sense of people's complaints about health care communication, not least in its negative, institutional forms. We know that institutional care encourages dependency, by means of both open (overt) and secret or disguised (covert) strategies on the part of care staff (Ryan and Scullion 2000). Although the situation is slowly changing, with a trend towards empowering users of health services, being a 'good patient' traditionally involves being passive, compliant and docile. The language of the nursing home is thought to be important in producing the disability itself. Moreover, despite the ethic of care in such institutions, the experience of being cared for is often profoundly dehumanising: 'Older residents must adapt to a new set of routines, expectations and rules, frequently compromising or abandoning their own lifetime preferences, habits and needs. Further, they must make these adaptations from the socially inferior or less powerful role of resident or patient' (Ryan *et al.* 1994, p. 238).

The examples of 'comfort talk' and 'secondary baby talk' in therapeutic encounters, alert us to the way that language is an act of socialisation in health care settings. Our talk may promote comfort and benefit individuals. Yet there is the potential for styles of communication, not least in patronising 'baby talk' that might incapacitate the client and place them in a position where they are disadvantaged and disabled. This should illustrate just how important it is that we reflect on language as action, thinking of it as a way of harming or healing those in our care.

Narratives of health and illness: the role of culture

The kinds of storylines or narratives that drive health care delivery and that we apply to people (as if they are characters in a drama) will tell us much about the possibilities and limitations of the care we deliver.

Our basic, fundamental ideas about medicine are embedded in culture and language such that most people today think that they know what a sick person is. However, history suggests that the way illness is defined in the twenty-first century depends a great deal on fairly recent changes in patterns of sickness and health. Everyday complaints like the common cold and gastrointestinal upsets have a set of symptoms that we expect to co-occur. As sufferers or healers, we tend to look for distinct patterns in illness. The illnesses we identify are different from those described in the eighteenth century; for example, we no longer claim to suffer from 'rising of the lights' (lung problems) or 'horseshoehead' (inflammation or water on the brain). Nevertheless, across the centuries, the coherence of an illness is an important part of the sufferer's experience of it.

The concern with narratives emerges from the everyday observation that much of our lived experience incorporates storytelling. When we meet someone for the first time we usually find out about them through an exchange of stories. Stories are important because they do not merely describe experience but constitute, construct, or, if you like, make it.

Nurses narrate both their own stories of care and the stories told to them by patients. This doesn't mean that the stories nurses or patients tell simply are fictional. What it does mean is that much of what happens between nurses and patients is to do with narration. This idea has been developed in psychology, sociology, anthropology and in the study of medical and nursing activities and the experiences of patients.

Reflective activity

Consider how much of your work depends on the stories you tell about yourself and about those for whom you care:

- How do you tell the story of your professional role? What is the story of being a nurse?
- How do the stories we tell about patients' problems influence the kind of care we make available to them?

In terms of the narratives of illness that nurses are likely to come across, it is important to consider the role that culture has in helping us to make sense of these phenomena and informing the story we build or construct. For people from European or North American white majority cultures, there will be a high degree of correspondence between the stories told by patients and professionals. This makes it much easier to take the signs, symptoms, syndromes and illnesses for granted. However, it is important to realise that such an understanding might be more difficult to obtain with people from different cultures to our own. The problems that people from such cultures express may seem to be at odds with dominant western medical notions of health and illness. Given that cross-cultural issues are becoming increasingly important in health care, as global migration changes the cultural map of the world (Choi 2002), we need to take the time and effort to consider cultural differences in the way people define or explain their illness states.

A good example of this kind of cultural difference in explanations can be found Sachs's (1983) account of Turkish women living in Sweden:

> In the forty days after childbirth known as the *lohusa* period, a woman is liable to contract *albasmasi*. This condition, characterised by the woman seeing everything in red, turning hot and getting cramps as well as choking, is one of the most feared reactions connected with childbirth. All women have heard of it and been in touch with it one way or another in Kulu (a region of Turkey). *Albasmasi* is an illness with specific symptoms. When a case has been established, it is only the personal and folk sectors of health care that can provide treatment. A scientific doctor will not be consulted. The Kulu women know that only their own experts can cure a person from *albasmasi* and that scientific doctors have not even heard of the illness.
>
> (Sachs 1983, p. 86)

In the case of this unusual or exotic complaint debate might revolve around the extent to which *albasmasi* is similar to postnatal depression, and therefore merely a cultural variation of a universal form of mental illness (see Carr and Vitaliano 1985). In addition, we might consider the benefits from the traditional treatment to be similar to the placebo effect or correspond with Euro-American concepts of psychotherapy.

However, for the practitioner confronted with a client who describes their problems in unfamiliar terms, it is often of secondary importance whether a 'better' approximation to their problems might be found in our western textbooks. There is a clear need for assessing the client in their own terms. This means that practitioners must explore other cultures, their ways of seeing and feeling, appreciating that other people might formulate or perceive reality in unfamiliar and surprising ways.

Reflective activity

Consider the comments of a woman of South Asian parentage speaking after her nephew had died in an accident: 'My heart is weak. I am ill with too much thinking . . . the blood becomes weaker with worry . . . I have the illness of sorrows' (Fenton and Sadiq-Sangster 1996)

● Can this account be repackaged as depression, or does labelling what she is suffering as depression lose some of the culturally important information which could lead to her being helped?

● Do existing forms, records, checklists that you use in your practice allow for the inclusion of such accounts? If not, why not?

● How could health care practice be broadened to include more of the experience of other cultures?

Another feature of human communication that is related to the way people give accounts of their illness, or the way they talk about their problems, is the use of metaphors: 'My flesh is *cotton wool*', 'I am in a *dark pit*', 'the pain is *hot*'. Migliore (1993) describes the way Sicilian-Canadians use the idea of *nerves* to 'express feelings of concern and distress over their social situation. They translate social problems into the metaphorical language of psychic [mental] and somatic [bodily] distress' (p. 343). 'Nerves' operates both as a sort of illness, and as a device for metaphorically expressing personal and social problems. These metaphors of illness may be especially powerful. Some theorists, such as Lakoff (1987) argue, even more radically, that **metaphor** influences not only how we perceive reality but that it can also structure how we experience that reality.

⌐ Keywords

Metaphor/metaphorical
When a word or phrase is applied imaginatively to something it does not literally resemble In order to emphasise particular qualities, for example 'You are a brick', 'He is a bag of nerves'

elleЯ**Refle****Reflective activity**

Read carefully the following lay and professional descriptions of psychiatric interventions from the 1970s:

(a) . . . deprivation of food, bed, walks in the open air, visitors, mail, or telephone calls; solitary confinement; deprivation of reading or entertainment materials; immobilising people by tying them into wet sheets and then exhibiting them to staff and other patients; other physical restraints on body movement; drugging the mind against the client's will; incarceration in locked wards; a range of public humiliations such as the prominent posting of alleged intentions to escape or commit suicide, the requirement of public confessions of misconduct or guilt, and public announcement of individual misdeeds and abnormalities. (Edelman 1974, p. 300)

(b) . . . discouraging sick behaviour and encouraging healthy behaviour through the selective granting of rewards; the availability of seclusion, restraints, and closed wards to grant a patient a respite from interaction with others and from making decisions, and prevent harm to himself or others; enabling him to think about his behaviour, to cope with his temptations to elope and succumb to depression, and to develop a sense of security; immobilising the patient to calm him, satisfy his dependency needs, give him the extra nursing attention he values, and enable him to benefit from peer confrontation; placing limits on his acting out; and teaching him that the staff cares (Edelman 1974, p. 302)

● List the ways in which the language used in these accounts differ.

● What can we learn about professional language from these different accounts?

In other words, we need to be especially sensitive to how the language and metaphors used by patients or clients *mean something to us*. Often our interpretations of what people *are saying* can be flawed. We may jump to the wrong conclusions. We might simply assume that a person means this or that. For example, we might consider that a person is in mental disorder if they say things like 'The electric is damaging my brain', 'I am God', 'There is a voice in my head telling me what to do.' But this may not be the case. It is therefore, important to allow people to explain, expand upon or put what they say into context.

Language crucially informs the way that diagnoses are achieved and 'progress' is accomplished. This has important implications for ethnic sensitivity in nursing practice, as the dominant understandings of progress or desirable outcomes in Euro-American medicine and psychiatry will not necessarily be shared by other cultures. Understanding the language of health care is important in making sense of the critiques of medicine and psychiatry offered from anti-racist or feminist positions, where mainstream medical and psychiatric care are argued to embody white, male, middle-class assumptions and values (Parker *et al.* 1995).

Reflective activity

Margaret is 38 years old and is suffering from systemic lupus erythematosus, a disorder of the connective tissues, primarily affecting women aged in their thirties and forties. It may involve arthritis, and problems with the kidneys, heart and brain. One day she opens up and begins to talk about her condition: 'If you have lupus, I mean one day it's my liver; one day it's my joints; one day it's my head, and it's like people really think you're a hypochondriac if you keep complaining about different ailments . . . It's like you don't want to say anything because people are going to start thinking, you know, "God, don't go near her, all she is . . . is complaining about this." And I think that's why I never say anything because I feel like everything I have is related one way or another to the lupus but most of the people don't know I have lupus, and even those that do are not going to believe that ten different ailments are the same thing. And I don't want anybody saying, you know, [that] they don't want to come around me because I complain' (adapted from Charnaz (1991, pp.114–115)

● How is Margaret making sense of her illness experience?

● Does Margaret's account fit with your own ideas of illness?

● How could Margaret tell others about it in a way that might make her life easier?

Thus, the ways in which the patient or client and his or her problems are formulated, may have important practical consequences for their future. In this respect, it is important that nurses remain vigilant about the potential for oppression in everyday health care language and communication, and the frameworks for understanding and problem solving which are embedded in everyday practice.

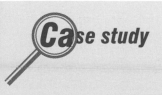

Case study

On a surgical ward, you find a male patient sitting up in bed, crying. Other staff members are engaged with various tasks or seem to ignore him. You know that the patient is recovering from a below-the-knee amputation and that he is struggling to come to terms with this loss, not least because he is a promising marathon runner. Earlier that day you were warned by the nurse in charge on the ward not to 'sit on beds talking to patients' because the 'ward is busy' and 'students need to learn what to do'. You believe that you should take time to interact with and emotionally support the patient. But first, you decide to clear things with the nurse in charge. What case would you make to the nurse in charge that you should spend time in conversation with the patient?

Key points · Top tips

- The way that people communicate will be affected by a variety of factors, not least age, gender, social class, culture and ethnicity
- People adopt different styles of speaking for different occasions
- We need to be aware that power – higher status and authority – is often demonstrated in communication
- Language can promote positive or negative outcomes
- Healthcare language can support particular political or ideological points of view
- Professional accounts or stories out healthcare shape and influence the kind of care that is delivered
- Patient narratives provide valuable insight into their experiences of health and illness

RRRRRRapid recap

Check your progress so far by working through each of the following questions:

1. What are the two key, basic models of communication?
2. Which area of the brain is involved in the production of speech?
3. What term is sometimes applied to the organisation and design of society according to particular viewpoints, norms or rules?
4. What special term can be used in reference to activities such as praising, warning, promising or apologising?
5. What do we call the patronising, child-like speech used with older adults considered frail?

If you have difficulty with more than one of the questions, read through the section again to refresh your understanding before moving on.

Over to you

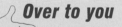

Read:

Crawford, P., Brown, B. and Nolan, P. (1998) *Communicating Care: The Language of Nursing*. Stanley Thornes, Cheltenham.

Hargie, P. and Dickson, D. (2004) *Skilled Interpersonal Communication: Research, Theory and Practice*, 4th edn. Routledge, London and New York.

References

Ambady, N., Koo, J., Rosxenthal, R. and Winograd, C.H. (2002) Physical therapists non-verbal communication predicts geriatric patients' health outcomes. *Psychology and Aging*, **17**(3), 443–452.

Bandura, A. (1986) *Social Foundations of Thought and Action: A social cognitive theory.* Prentice-Hall, Englewood Cliffs, NJ.

Bennett, B. (1996) How nurses in a stroke rehabilitation unit attempt to meet the psychological needs of patients who become depressed following a stroke. *Journal of Advanced Nursing*, **23**(2): 314–321.

Bradshaw, J. (1998) Assessing and intervening in the communication environment. *British Journal of Learning Disabilities*, **26**(2), 62–66.

Bricher, G. (1999) Paediatric nurses, children and the development of trust. *Journal of Clinical Nursing*, **8**, 451–458.

Cantwell, J. (2000) Pressures, priorities and pre-emptive practice. *Speech and Language Therapy*, Winter, 16–19.

Caporael, L., Lukaszewski, M. and Culbertson, G. (1983) Secondary baby talk: Judgements by institutionalised elderly and their caregivers. *Journal of Personality and Social Psychology*, **44**(4), 746–754.

Caris-Verhallen, W.M.C.M., de Gruitjer, I.M., Kerkstra, A. and Bensing, J. (1999) Factors related to nurse communication with elderly people. *Journal of Advanced Nursing*, **30**(5), 1106–1117.

Carr, J.E. and Vitaliano, P.P. (1985) The theoretical implications of converging research on depression and the culture bound syndromes (eds Kleinman, A. and Good, B.). In: *Culture and Depression.* Los Angeles: University of California Press.

Charnaz, K. (1991) *Good Days, Bad Days: The self in chronic illness and time.* Rutgers University Press, New Brunswick, NJ.

Choi, H. (2002) Understanding adolescent depression in ethnocultural context. *Advances in Nursing Science*, **25**(2), 71–85.

Chomsky, N. (1976) *Reflections on Language.* Fontana, London.

Crawford, P., Brown, B. and Nolan, P. (1998) *Communicating Care: The language of nursing.* Stanley Thornes, Cheltenham.

Department of Health (2003) *Essence of Care: Benchmarks for communication between patients, carers and health care personnel.* Department of Health, London.

de Wilde, I. and de Bot, K. (1989) Taal van verzorgenden tegen ouderen in een psychogeriatrisch verpleeghuis (A simplified speech register in caregivers' speech to elderly demented patients). *Tijdschrift voor Gerontologie en Geriatrie*, **20**, 97–100.

Dimitrovsky, L., Spector, H., Levy-Shiff, R. and Vakil, E. (1998) Interpretation of facial expressions of affect in children with learning disabilities with verbal or non-verbal deficits. *Journal of Learning Disabilities*, **31**(3), 286–292.

Dumble, M. and Tuson, W. (1998) Identifying eating and drinking difficulties. *Speech and Language Therapy Practice*, Winter, 4–6.

Edelman, M. (1974) The political language of the helping professions. *Politics and Society*, **4**, 295–310.

Erber, N.P. and Scherer, S.C. (1999) Sensory loss and communicative difficulties in the elderly. *Australian Journal on Ageing*, **18**(1), 4–9.

Fairclough, N. (1989) *Language and Power.* Longman, London.

Fenton, S. and Sadiq-Sangster, A. (1996) Culture, relativism, and the expression of mental distress: South Asian women in Britain. *Sociology of Health and Illness*, **18**(1) 66–85.

Hargie, P. and Dickson, D. (2004) *Skilled Interpersonal Communication: Research, theory and practice*, 4th edn. Routledge, London and New York.

Hemsley, B., Sigafoos, J., Balandin S., Forbes, R., Taylor C., Green, V.A. and Parmenter, T. (2001) Nursing the patient with severe communication impairment. *Journal of Advanced Nursing* **35**(6) 827–835.

Jakobson, R. (1960) Closing statement: linguistics and poetics. In: Style in Language (ed. Sebeok, T.A.). Massachusetts: MIT Press, pp. 350–377.

Lakoff, G., (1987) *Women, Fire and Dangerous Things: What categories reveal about the mind.* University of Chicago Press, Chicago.

Larkin, K.T., Martin, R.R. and McClain, S.E. (2002) Cynical hostility and the accuracy of decoding facial expressions of emotions. *Journal of Behavioural Medicine*, **25**(3), 285–293.

Mathieson, C.M. and Stam, H.J. (1995) Re-negotiating identity: Cancer narratives. *Sociology of Health and Illness* **17**(3): 283–306.

Migliore. S. (1993) "Nerves": The role of metaphor in the cultural framing of experience. *Journal of Contemporary Ethnography*, **22**(3), 331–360.

Parker, I., Georgaca, E., Harper, D., McLaughlin, T. and Stowell-Smith, M. (1995) *Deconstructing Psychopathology.* Sage Publications Inc, London and Thousand Oaks, CA.

Pell, M.D. (2002) Evaluation of non-verbal emotion in face and voice: Some preliminary findings on a new battery of tests. *Brain and Cognition*, **48**(2–3), 499–504.

Pinker, S. (1994) *The language Instinct.* W. Morrow & Co, New York.

Potter, J. (1996) *Representing Reality*. Sage, London.

Pound, P., Bury, M., Gompertz, P. and Ebrahim, S. (1995) Stroke patients' views on their admission to hospital. *British Medical Journal*, **311**, 18–22.

Pound, P., Sabin, C. and Ebrahim, S. (1999) Observing the process of care: A stroke unit, elderly care unit and general medical ward compared. *Age and Ageing*, **28**, 433–440.

Proctor, A., Morse, J.M. and Khonsari, E.S., (1996) Sounds of comfort in the trauma centre: How nurses talk to patients in pain. *Social Science and Medicine*, **42**(12), 1669–1680.

Ratzan, S.C., Payne, J.G. and Bishop, C. (1996) The status and scope of health communication. *Journal of Heath Communication*, **1**, 25–41.

Reid, S.A. and Ng, S.H. (1999) Language, power and intergroup relations. *Journal of Social Issues*, **55**, 119–139.

Robillard, A. B. (1996) Anger in the social order. *Body and Society*, **2**(1), 17–30.

Ryan, A.A. and Scullion, H.S. (2000) Family and staff perceptions of the role of families in nursing homes. *Journal of Advanced Nursing*, **32**(2), 626–634.

Ryan E.B., Meredith, S.D. and Shantz, G.B. (1994) Evaluative perceptions of patronising speech addressed to institutionalised elders in contrasting conversational contexts. *Canadian Journal on Ageing*, **13**(2), 236–248.

Sachs, L. (1983) *Evil Eye or Bacteria: Turkish migrant women and Swedish health care.* Stockholm studies in social anthropology: University of Stockholm.

Searle, J. (1979) *Speech Acts: An essay in the philosophy of language*. Cambridge University Press, London.

Shannon, C.E. and Weaver, W. (1949) *A Mathematical Model of Communication.* University of Illinois Press, Urbana, IL.

Sumner J. (2001) Caring in nursing: A different interpretation. *Journal of Advanced Nursing*, **35**(6), 926–932.

Sundin, K. and Jansson, L. (2003) Understanding and being understood as a creative caring phenomenon in care of patients with stroke and aphasia. *Journal of Clinical Nursing*, **12**, 107–116.

Sundin, K., Norberg, A. and Jansson, L. (2001) The meaning of skilled care providers' relationships with stroke and aphasia patients. *Qualitative Health Research*, **11**(3), 308–321.

Tye-Murray, N. and Schum, L. (1994) Conversation training for frequent communication partners. *Journal of the Academy of Rehabilitative Audiology*, **27**, 209–222.

2

Basic interpersonal verbal and non-verbal skills

Learning outcomes

By the end of this chapter you should be able to:

- Understand the importance, use and value of basic interpersonal skills
- Identify key verbal and non-verbal aspects of communication.

Demonstrating basic interpersonal skills

In this section we examine a range of verbal and non-verbal skills that you will need to think about to improve the way you communicate not only with the patients you work with but also their relatives and your fellow professionals. The skills you need from the moment you first meet a new patient, through to some of the times when they may want to share some of their worries with you, will be examined and discussed in this chapter.

Verbal and non-verbal communication

As we shall see, there is a wide range of verbal and non-verbal communication activity such as eye contact, nodding, smiling, friendly or humorous small-talk or phatic communication, touch, facial, hand or body gestures that are vital in establishing and sustaining rapport with other people. These can be seen as ordinary yet essential aspects of creating, sustaining and terminating therapeutic relationships with patients/clients – and often they can be done while carrying out other tasks and duties.

Verbal communication is a diverse and complex activity. How we speak or write about patients and clients – the words we use – will say much about the kind of care we are giving. Are we polite? Do we use dignified language? How do we portray others in the language we use? Again, we would be concerned with the pitch, tone or pace of our spoken language. Do these fit the occasion or situation we are in? For example, a higher pitch of voice can convey that we are interested and engaged with another person (Argyle 1994). A particular voice tone or inflection might convey warmth or hostility for example, even flirting. The pace at which we speak may convey lack of time, or mood. We might speak fast if we are happy or enthusiastic, but much slower if we are feeling low or depressed. We would also need to consider the

Keywords

Jargon
Specialist words or phrases used by professionals

kind of vocabulary that we use, whether we use **jargon** or plain, easily understood expressions, etc.

Aside from spoken or written verbal language, a key aspect of all communication is the way we use non-verbal or body language. By our gestures, postures and facial expressions, we are able to convey rich and varied messages to other people. For example, there are approximately 20,000 different facial expressions. When combined with other gestures and movements, there could be around 700,000 kinds of non-verbal display.

Non-verbal communication involves a variety of issues. On the one hand its functions can be relational, that is, demonstrate how we feel towards others. Our facial expressions, gestures and postures might express whether we like or dislike the other person, wish to dominate or control them, or engage intimately. Non-verbal expression can be used to regulate our interactions with other people by signalling that we are about to end a turn of conversation or desire to say something. They may help attaining a goal, such as pointing at the thing we want, amplifying what we say, e.g. punching the air with a celebratory 'Yes!' when we hear favourable news or holding up the palm of a hand when we don't want someone to come closer. Sometimes, of course, we say things such as 'I'm OK' when our facial expression, gestures and posture tell a very different story! At other times, our non-verbal communication can simply be distracting or irritating, as with **mannerisms**. Mannerisms can be very distracting in communications, and should be avoided. Fidgeting, tapping, or doodling, for example, broadcast that you are not sufficiently interested or engaged with another person.

Keywords

Mannerism
A habitual movement or gesture

Reflective activity

- Place yourself in front of a mirror and rehearse as many combined facial expressions, gestures and postures as you can
- Identify what the expressions might mean
- Try to make all three kinds of non-verbal behaviour convey the same meaning. Then use gestures or posture that do not fit with your facial expression, for example, smiling warmly while shaking your fist or crossing your arms
- Try signalling that you are cold or uncaring
- Now try signalling that you are warm and approachable
- On a scale of 1–10 (with 1 'appears cold' and 10 'appears warm') what score do you think patients or clients would award you?
- Finally, how might non-verbal communications amplify what you say? Or how might they be at odds with your comments?

Other important non-verbal communication occurs through images, symbols and drawing.

Images and symbols

Modern society is 'information rich' with a wide range of communication, not least through an expanding media with all kinds of images and symbols bombarding us – whether in signs, advertisements, film, television, photography or art. Most of us use a wide spectrum of all these forms of communication in addition to verbal/spoken and written language. In healthcare we use **images** and **symbols** widely to promote healthy lifestyles, provide information and enhance the quality of the environment.

Keywords

Image
Representation of a person or thing in sculpture, painting, or on screen

Symbol
A mark or character taken as an agreed sign for an object, idea, process or function, e.g. skull and crossbones to indicate poison, or a simple stick man on a door to indicate entry to a male toilet

Reflective activity

- What use is made of symbols or images in providing care to patients?
- List the ways in which symbols or images could be used to improve communication with patients

Drawing or graphical communication

Drawings can prove useful in communication in health settings. For example, it may be especially useful when communicating with people from different language groups or with people who suffer sensory or communicative impairments. As Rao (1995) notes there are cases of people who have been severely communication-impaired following a stroke becoming functional communicators once more through drawing. Other authors have also noted the way that drawings can provide insight into the emotional lives of children who have suffered a traumatic event (Clements *et al.* 2001; Wellings 2001).

Key points   Top tips

- How we speak or write about patients and clients – the words we use – will say much about the kind of care we are giving
- A key aspect of all communication is the way we use non-verbal or body language
- By our gestures, postures and facial expressions, we are able to convey rich and varied messages to other people
- Non-verbal communication can be relational, demonstrating how we feel about others
- Non-verbal signals may either mirror or be at odds with feelings or emotions
- We need to tune-in or tailor our communication to suit the preferred communication styles or channels of others that may involve images, symbols, drawing

Core interpersonal skills

The following sections indicate some of the core interpersonal skills that promote a healthy communicative environment for both healthcare staff and patients. We must remember that nurses already bring to their work a wealth of communicating experience from their lives outside the healthcare setting, and are also developing their knowledge of how to communicate in various contexts by being with and learning from their peers and expert clinicians. The overview that follows acknowledges that in these ways nurses are already skilled communicators but aims to re-emphasise just how important some basic forms of communication are, such as smiling or greeting people. It does not set out in stone what should or should not be done – after all it is not possible, for example, to say exactly how much eye contact or touch we should use in our interactions – nor is it a comprehensive 'cook book' or guide. This section identifies the potential benefits of particular styles or approaches in communication, and advances the view that these should be used to the maximum effect in clinical settings. Doing this will require an honest and ongoing self reflection and assessment of the following: how we communicate individually; what should stand as appropriate use of interpersonal skills; the evidence that supports our choices in how we interact with people in clinical settings; and the constraints or limitations that healthcare organisations and environments place on this activity. In the final chapter of the book, we will develop some of these ideas further in suggesting a model that emphasises brief, ordinary and effective healthcare communication.

Making yourself approachable

Making yourself approachable and available to patients or service users, their carers or relatives, and your colleagues and other carers from statutory and non-statutory services such as social work, voluntary agencies and so on is of vital importance.

The terms 'approachable' and 'available' can be considered to be very close in their meaning. Think about how you can make yourself approachable to the range of people mentioned above. An important issue is your own personal **boundaries** and space. The way you make yourself approachable to your partner, or best friend, compared to a service user or a fellow professional can be very different. Why is that and how do you do it while still retaining a sense of personal and professional honesty and integrity?

⚷ *Keywords*

Boundary/boundaries
Limits, both physical, in terms of space, and what you may and may not do as a professional carer

elleЯ*Reflective activity*

Think how you make yourself 'approachable' to the range of different people you meet during the course of your working day:

- How effective are you at doing this?
- How do you change in relation to the person you meet?
- How might you do it a little better?

Smiling

While LaFrance and Hecht (1999) point out that smiling is a key form of expression that can have a number of meanings, it tends to indicate that you like or are positive towards another person (Argyle 1994), and promotes attraction or likeability (Monahan 1998). As such, it is one of the most important brief communications that a health professional can cultivate and something that can be easily achieved in the busiest of clinical areas. As Duggan and Parrott (2001) found, smiling strongly indicates attentive listening and encourages disclosure.

There is another good reason for health professionals to indulge in smiling. Evidence suggests you may be able to improve your mood by smiling! This is based on the facial feedback hypothesis that 'facial expression affects emotional expression and behavior' (Davis and Pallidino 2000).

In addition to smiling, there are other expressions and gestures that can be deployed briefly to good effect in communication in health settings. For example, head nods and eyebrow raises can be a potent means of showing that you are an active and interested listener (Rosenfeld and Hancks 1980). Simply winking or raising a hand may convey that you are acknowledging the presence of another person.

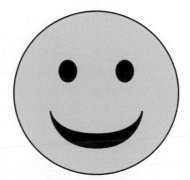

Figure 2.1 *Why am I so popular?*

Top tips

Often a smile is all you need to start your effective nursing work, but make sure that your smile is suitable for what is going on around you!

Welcoming, greeting and ordinary conversation

As Holli and Calabrese (1998) note, greetings that open communication are vitally important. Alongside other techniques, such as direct eye contact and smiling (see below), the use of welcoming or greeting remarks result in increased levels of customer satisfaction (Brown and Sulzerazaroff 1994). They may be accompanied by touch (see below), for example, in handshaking, and at their most positive they convey an atmosphere for continued interaction.

Greetings are often simple, such as 'Hi', 'Hello' or 'How are you?', which will tend to draw simple, and sometimes matched responses. In terms of the latter, one tends to expect fairly neutral responses: 'Fine', 'Pretty good', 'Okay', etc. Although, in clinical settings, one might expect more direct and reality-based disclosure, such as 'Not so good', 'I'm still getting pain', 'I've been better'. Such brief remarks may provide useful assessment information for the sensitive practitioner to pursue further, or at least result in a minimal but positive show of sympathy

This is where it all starts for you and the patient. The style in which you carry out the first contact with them sets the tone for at least that occasion and maybe for future ones as well. It is essential to acknowledge the person with whom you have just come into contact, in a respectful and professional way.

Reflective activity

Imagine that you are the nurse in charge on a medical ward and the patient arrives with a relative. They are being admitted for a series of investigations at the suggestion of their GP:

How would you greet them in an appropriate way?

What is it that you hope to achieve in the next few minutes?

How do think the patient may be feeling?

How do think their relative may be feeling?

How quickly do you form a first impression of the patient?

How quickly do they form an impression of you?

Does this matter, and if so, why?

Keywords

Demeanour
The way you look and behave together with your attitude

Keywords

Intention
What you are deliberately aiming to do as a professional carer

Probably the most widely useable presentation or demeanour would be one of neutral friendliness. This, of course would be altered according to the situation at the time or the quality of your relationship with the patient. For example, your **demeanour** would be very different if you were breaking the news of her father's death to a middle-aged woman, compared to how you would look when you were admitting a child to your ward, who needed an emergency procedure carrying out.

What could some of the possible differences be in the nurse's presentation during these two scenarios? Again, the conversation between the nurse and the patient will vary greatly in its content but as a result of the nurse's deliberate **intention**, not just a random happening. This is guided by a combination of the care plan objectives and consideration of what the patient needs on an immediate basis.

In the case of the recently bereaved daughter, for example, the conversation would probably open by the nurse preparing the recipient for the bad news that follows: 'Hello Mrs James. Please, take a seat. I'm afraid things took a turn for the worse. I'm sorry but I've got some bad news for you.' Here the nurse is very quickly trying to prepare the relative for the shock (maybe) that is to come. (In the event of breaking the news, people, of course have very different reactions. The experienced nurse will be exposed to responses and behaviours that are quite unexpected, sometimes.)

Compare this to the nurse who is admitting the child: 'Hiya Jenny, Let's pop you onto this bed so we can have a proper look at you. I see you've brought your doll to help us out. Good! Mum, you can stay with her if you want to?' The nurse who is thinking about maximising the effect of his or her conversational impact on the nursing intervention will be considerate of most of the following: pace, tone, pitch (in terms of the kind of language used as in the examples above), volume, avoiding jargon (unless it's helpful to use it).

There are also occasions when the situation is best served by an introductory preamble. This is a piece of ordinary conversation that leads up to the real nursing intervention. In the above examples, in very different ways the nurse is addressing the 'business' of nursing very quickly, within a small number of sentences. This is deliberate. In the following example the nurse is visiting an elderly lady about whom the GP has expressed some concerns. She takes a little longer to get to the 'business' – but she still does. There is a reason for this – it is a deliberate intention of the nurse to do it this way: 'Hello again, Edith. Thanks for agreeing to see me again so soon. It's a bit cold out there isn't it? Aren't the nights drawing in again? Yes I would *love* a cup of tea. Has your daughter been in touch lately? How's her son getting on at school now? I've got the results of those tests you had at the hospital – do you remember, your GP said they'd take about a month. But they've come back much quicker than usual. Anyway, sit down because I need to go through some of these results with you Edith.' You will note that in the 'chit chat' the nurse has tentatively tested some aspects of her patient:

1. Is she orientated to the time of year/change of seasons?
2. Is her daughter (Edith's only support) still in touch with Edith?
3. Can she manage to make a cup of tea appropriately and safely?
4. Does she remember going to hospital, for the tests?

This all takes place as part of an opening 'chat', but as you can see, even this has the intention of quickly re-assessing (and thus helping) the patient.

Reflective activity

Think about the last few occasions when patients have been admitted to your work area:
How did they seem?
Were they worried, upset, relieved, anxious, pleased?
How did you and your colleagues respond to the 'mood' of these patients?
What seemed to help?
What did not seem to help?

Keywords

Phatic conversation
Ordinary conversation that enhances social fellowship

Such 'chit chat', 'small talk' or what has been called **phatic conversation** is something we all use on a daily basis, commenting on the weather, perhaps, or other 'light' subject matter. It is basically, as Malinowski (1922) put it, 'language used in free, aimless, social intercourse'. Yet as we indicate above it can be very useful in achieving specific goals in our work with patients. Most importantly, as Burnard (2003) notes, such 'small talk' can help to develop a rapport with patients and clients, presenting no threat and encouraging further disclosure that may provide key opportunities in negotiating care with an individual. In fact, as Brown and Levinson (1987) argue 'the subject of talk is not as important as the fact of carrying on a conversation that is amply loaded with . . . markers of emotional agreement'. It promotes a feeling of equality and belonging. If you don't believe that the form of conversation is more important than the content or meaning of the transaction try to recall in detail what you talked about in conversations you had two weeks ago . . . last week . . . or even yesterday!

Top tips

Key points

Think about how you present yourself to patients. This has a major influence on how effectively you are able to nurse them. It is preferable that the patients you work with at least feel comfortable and safe with you, before anything else.

Remember that it is important that you are aware of the balance of the conversational weighting. The aim should be for the majority of the talking to be done by the patient, and the majority of the listening to be done by the nurse. The exception might be if you were taking on the temporary role of advising or giving information when, of course, the weighting reverses. In this instance, you do the talking and the patient does the listening. However, you quickly reverse roles again when you carefully check that the patient has actually heard, and understands, what you have just said to them!

Here is an example:

Nurse: So, John, are you nearly ready to go? Have you collected your medication?

John: Yes, I'm all fixed up. Sandie should be here soon to pick me up.

Nurse: I bet she's thrilled to bits to have you home again?

John: That's right. I did wonder if this day would ever come around. I feel like I've lost a big part of my life in here.

Nurse: Yes, I remember you got really down at one point didn't you?

John: Still, you lot got me through it. If it wasn't for everyone here I'm not sure I would have made it. It's funny, in some ways I'll miss the people I've met here.

Nurse: Well, you know where we are. You will remember to take plenty of fluids with that medication won't you? You remember the pharmacist stressing that, don't you? You have the appointment card in your wallet as well. Don't forget that it's essential to come to the follow-up appointments. So we'll see you in a month?

John: Got it!

Here, in what seems to be a straightforward conversation, the nurse has checked that John has the essentials he needs just prior to discharge. She has clarified an important item regarding his medication. She briefly validates his feelings about the time he has spent in hospital. She has re-checked that he understands the importance of this, and the significance of his post-discharge recall visits. She deliberately uses accentuated words like 'stressing' and 'essential'. Throughout, the tone of the conversation is positive and upbeat.

Top tips
In situations such as the one above, where you are giving important information to patients (or relatives), the language you use is important. As in the situation above, words like *essential*, *critical*, *very important*, can cut through some of the distractions that patients experience when under stress.   If you are still doubtful that the patient has heard and taken in what you've said, consider writing the information down.

Naming

We know that naming and forms of address have been an important part of communication down the ages. Across different cultures there are various naming ceremonies and people gather their notion of selfhood and identity in terms of their names. Their names may link them to families, religious beliefs, or indicate a variety of other affiliations. A person's name is important to them, and we know that the appropriate use of a patient's or client's name in communication leads to positive evaluation of the professional (Hargie *et al* 1999) That said, it is important to use names appropriately. This may mean, for example, addressing an individual by a formal name such as 'Mr Johnson' and only using informal first name terms if the patient wants you to.

Politeness

A fundamental aspect of communication, which helps to create and maintain interpersonal relationships, is politeness. We all value politeness in our interactions with other people and this can be signalled through balanced, shared conversation with appropriate turn-taking and a willingness to use words and phrases that convey apology for intrusion, gratitude or to save people's 'face'. For example, we might reduce the discomfort of intrusion into an individual's world of thoughts and feelings by using rather tentative phrases that invite rather than demand information, such as 'Would you be able to tell me . . .' or 'Do you think you could say a little bit more about . . .'

Top tips

To be polite you must:

- invite rather than demand information
- use words and phrases such as 'please' and 'thank you'
- avoid interrupting
- strive to protect, repair or bolster the 'face', self-value or self-worth of others
- be tentative or apologetic in initiating talk or discussion about delicate topics or issues
- reduce the impact of uncomfortable or embarrassing intrusions or interventions

Using dignified or self-respecting language

As a professional it is essential that you, at all times, aspire to behave in a professional (and thus dignified) way. A significant part of this dignity comes from your actions and the language that accompanies them. Your dignity as a professional should be maintained regardless of the clinical setting you work in, and the age or gender of your patients. The 'pitch' of it may be modified somewhat depending on circumstances. For example, consider the way that the paediatric nurse behaves, interacting with a six-year-old girl who is due to have minor surgery, and how this might be different from that of the nurse working with the unpredictable and sometimes aggressive 'challenging behaviour' older adult in a mental health setting. The spoken language and non-verbal communication used by each nurse may be strikingly different. What is certain is that the professional nurse will have their own way of behaving in a dignified self-respecting way that you will be able to see always, as a consistent part of their nursing.

Reflective activity

How do the nurses you work with, demonstrate a dignified and self-respecting approach?

What do they say to patients?

How do they treat patients?

Praising

When we receive words of praise from people it makes us feel good or positive about ourselves and tends to motivate us to repeat particular kinds of behaviour. This is similar in health settings. We know that the use of compliments, praise and approval increases patient satisfaction with care and compliance with care interventions (Holli and Calabrese 1998).

Humour

Humour is a powerful aspect of communication. It is a key factor in promoting engagement and rapport with others. You will know from life experience that humour is a good way to get to know someone – it's a great connector. For example at school, in your family, in social situations and other work situations, it is very likely that your fondest experiences and memories will be connected to situations where in some way humour played a part. Just as humour can serve to enhance easy and enjoyable situations, it can also consolidate fragile situations, and diffuse difficult situations. The value of humour in health settings has a long history and its benefits are supported by anecdotal evidence from clinicians themselves. Various commentators and patients themselves have considered laughter or the use of appropriate, sensitive humour as a healing or therapeutic activity and research has shown physiological and psychological benefits, for example, in terms of reducing the levels of stress hormones, enhancing the immune system and the release of the body's natural painkillers or endorphins. It is also considered as a key activity in developing a friendly relationship with others.

In the professional nursing setting, humour plays an important role as a stress reliever, and partnership and team bonding agent. This is the enhancing side of humour. Its aspect as a consolidator can be seen when a tense situation is being experienced.

Difficult situations are a very regular occurrence in nursing, and some clinical settings seem to experience a higher rate of difficult situations than others, of course. Where appropriate, the use of humour can ease the return to a rather more relaxed atmosphere after a difficult shift or a difficult incident. Each clinical area seems to develop its own culture of humour, some of which would seem strange, or even inappropriate to an 'outsider'. It is clear, however, that this culture of humour can be very supportive to the professional nurses who understand it, and use it with sensitivity.

Over to you

Read:

Martin R.A. (2001) Humor, laughter, and physical health: Methodological issues and research findings. *Psychological Bulletin,* **127** (4), 504–519.

Mutual gaze/eye contact

Keywords

Mutual gaze

The exchange, return or reciprocation of eye contact

During interaction in contemporary Western cultures people typically spend about 60 per cent of the time gazing generally at one another (face, nose, mouth, etc.) and these gazes typically last about 3 seconds. Direct eye contact or **mutual gaze** take up 30 per cent of the time, with this more specific form of gaze lasting about 1 second.

It is with our eyes making contact with others that we truly make someone else feel visible. Balanced, appropriate eye contact is vital to ensuring the individuals feel responded to and involved in dialogue or conversation. This can be seen particularly clearly in maternal bonding in childhood and, as with touch, it is something that women make greater use of than men.

Crucially we tend to lengthen our eye-contact in positive interaction with others to convey our commitment and interest in them. While this is something that is deemed to increase satisfaction (see Brown and Sulzerazaroff 1994), such gaze always needs to be carefully judged so that the receiver does not feel stared at – something that may cause discomfort or simply be deemed impolite or threatening. When gaze is avoided by a health practitioner a patient or client may feel rejected and invisible. In essence, eye contact is something that tells us much about another person's emotions, attitudes, mental activity. It signals where we are in a relationship with other people, opens and closes our communication and assists in giving and receiving feedback.

The strange thing about eye contact is that often it is appropriate when you don't notice it. In the instances when it could be inappropriate (usually from your point of view) it is often because you notice it. For instance, when you are talking with someone who looks away from you, or at the ground, you may be tempted to draw conclusions from this. For example: is the other person shy or embarrassed, avoiding the issue you want to talk about, or being in some way dishonest? What if they stare straight at you with an unbroken gaze? Are they being hostile towards you? Do they find you fascinating in some unusual way? What if they look over your shoulder when you are talking? Have they seen something or someone more interesting than you? Are you boring them? Any of the above inferences or assumptions could be correct or incorrect. One way of starting to get a little nearer to understanding what is happening is to ask, if you can:

Nurse: You seem to be distracted by something over there John?
John: I was looking for my Dad. He's coming to collect me any time now. Sorry.

Or

John: I feel ill. I think I'm going to faint. Can I sit down?

Or

John: I don't want to talk about this now. It's too soon.

Reflective activity

What other versions of John's responses can you construct, given his 'inappropriate' eye contact with you?
   Think of an occasion where you felt uncomfortable because of someone's eye contact with you.
      How did the situation resolve?

Proximity

Proximity
Level of physical closeness to others

Keywords

Proxemics
The study or appreciation of this physical closeness

Our use of body space or **proximity** – that is, how close we position ourselves to others – will affect how messages are sent and received. You can sometimes make a reasonably accurate judgement as to the type of relationship between two or more people if you look at the distance at which they choose to position themselves from each other. You will see that people who have a formal 'professional' type of relationship will tend to be further away from each other than, for instance a couple who have a more intimate connection (Adler and Towne 1999). Their proximity (see **proxemics**) can be markedly different. This is likely to be emphasised also by the accompanying body language or non-verbal signals. For example, the 'professional' couple may stand or sit more than an arm's length apart and you may see indications such as arms folded, the use of barriers such as desks, crossed legs, a hand covering part of a face, and so on.

The more intimate couple are likely to sit or stand more closely, use much longer periods of eye contact (gaze) and perhaps use more personal non-verbal signals such as touch, and the more inviting uncrossed arms and legs. Barriers are likely to be noticeable by their absence. As has been noted before, however, it is important not to assume that lack of barriers means intimacy and great distance means cool professionalism.

Often when males are about to fight, the distance between them becomes inappropriately close, although again, there are often explicit non-verbal indicators such as finger pointing and aggressive posturing. The effective nurse will always attempt to clarify exactly what is happening.

Another factor which the thoughtful nurse would take into account is some reference to the culture, for the proximity between two or more people. It is noted that some cultural differences may cause people to position themselves at distances that may look inappropriate to you, i.e. much closer than you would expect, or much further apart.

Also do not forget that other factors, such as physical or mental illness, may have some influence on the proxemics of an interaction between two or more people. A deaf person may stand nearer you to lip read or hear you more clearly. A person who is in a state of mental disinhibition may also place themselves uncomfortably near to you.

Reflective activity

When you are next at work, note how people position themselves, in relation to each other.

Does their positioning depend on status, gender, authority, or emotional state? Or something else?

Top tips

If in doubt, keep your distance at first from patients and other people who you meet as a professional nurse. Get a little closer as you become more familiar and have a greater understanding of what is going on. This need not take very long – sometimes a few minutes or less. Many people in our culture are uncomfortable with, or are likely to misinterpret, premature closeness.

Posture

The shape or posture that we adopt with our bodies is enormously important and can be manipulated to the benefit of patients and clients. During conversation it is particularly important to use body posture, alongside facial expressions and gestures that mirror or

o—ᴉᴉ Keywords

Empathy

Ability to identify oneself with another person or 'step into their shoes'

reflect those of the person we are communicating with. It advances or signals **empathy** and promotes the sharing of their feelings. In fact, many of the strategies for positioning our bodies in relation to others are simple and briefly achieved.

Traditionally, one of the ways that new practitioners in health settings have remembered to use appropriate posture and non-verbal presentation when seated or standing is through the acronym SOLER (see Box 2.1). Although this is a bit simplistic, it is a useful reminder to get us thinking about how we are positioning our bodies in relation to other people. For people brought up in the UK, or in a Western culture, an appropriate non-verbal approach to communicating with patients should include facing them directly or *squarely* (not turning away) where possible in an *open posture* (not crossing your arms or curling up into a ball!). It is important to remember just how arm-crossing can appear hostile, defensive or convey that you are simply not interested in what a person has to say. *Lean forwards* slightly – again to show your personal commitment and interest. If you pull your head and shoulders back or stand or sit too far away, the patient may feel you are rejecting them or that they are in some way objectionable. Use regular but not fixed *eye contact*, and maintain a *relaxed* appearance or demeanour.

Box 2.1: SOLER

S   Face people **Squarely**
O   Maintain an **Open** shape to the body
L   **Lean** forward slightly
E   Use appropriate **Eye contact**
R   **Relax**

Posture can also give the observant nurse an important clue as to how someone may be feeling at a particular time. For example, you notice that one of your colleagues is slouching over a cup of tea in the office. You observe that usually she is more upright in her posture. Her appearance today is not usual for her and may reflect an unusual (for her) set of circumstances:

You: Fiona, you look a bit worse for wear this morning. Are you OK?
Fiona: I suppose so. I had a late night. I'm still struggling with that assignment I told you about. And I'm starting a cold. I'm thinking of packing it all in.

This statement seems to have confirmed some of what you may have suspected anyway. On the other hand:

You: Fiona, are you OK?

Fiona: Yeah, I'm fine. But I think the milk in this tea might be a bit 'off' and I was dying for a cuppa.

It's always a good idea to clarify how someone looks if it is important to you. Sometimes you will be surprisingly accurate, sometimes you won't. It's usually worth making the effort to ask, however, as long as you can avoid being over-intrusive.

Finally, since a great deal of record keeping is electronic, it is important to make some fundamental postural adjustments in communicating with patients when using computer terminals during consultations with patients. Here, the Calgary Cambridge Guide to help doctors develop rapport and involve patients when using computers during consultations (based on Kurtz *et al.* 1998, Silverman *et al.* 1998, and Kurtz *et al.* 2003) is useful for similar nurse-patient interactions. Box 2.2 provides a summary of key approaches adapted from their webpage (see below).

Box 2.2: Adapted Calgary Cambridge Guide for using computers during consultations

If the nurse is using the computer, she should:

- Do this in a way that does not disrupt the dialogue or rapport
- Adapt her behaviour to take into account her position relative to the patient and computer
- Maintain an open posture (not be hunched over the keyboard)
- Signpost (verbally or non-verbally) to indicate when attention is being paid to the computer screen. This is best done in natural breaks in the conversation and achieved by reaching for the mouse, turning towards the computer or using phrases such as: 'Just give me a minute while I look at the computer'' or 'Forgive me while I look at the screen' or 'There is some information I need, I just need a moment to find it'
- Control the structure of the consultation in order to reduce the likelihood of the patient talking when looking at the screen
- Respond to the patient's non-verbal signals when attending to the computer
- Involve the patient in the process by explaining why she is using the computer
- If the computer is being used as an information source, negotiate the use of such information with the patient
- Let the patient read information from the screen when appropriate

Again, adapting slightly the Calgary Cambridge guide, there are three main options for arranging seating around the desk/computer that will require the nurse to adopt different communication styles. Each of these options has advantages and disadvantages, although the third option appears to offer the best compromise.

Option 1: computer screen and patient at opposite ends of the desk

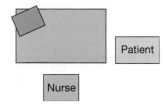

Advantages
- Easy for the patient to see the screen
- Easy for the patient to determine whether nurse's attention is on them or the screen.

Disadvantages
- The nurse may appear to be cutting off the patient when she turns to the screen
- When looking at the screen the nurse will not be able to pick up on the patient's non-verbal communication
- Rapport needs to be re-established after the nurse turns back from the screen
- Possibility of 'third party' information being seen by the patient.

Option 2: computer screen and patient at same end of the desk

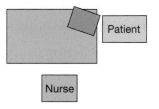

Advantages
- The nurse can view screen without turning her head or body away
- Easier to observe and respond to patient's non-verbal communication.

Disadvantages
- The patient may be unsure whether the nurse is looking at them or the screen
- Difficult for the patient to view the screen if required.

Option 3: computer screen in middle of desk

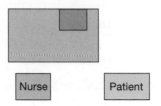

Nurse   Patient

Advantages
- More open arrangement
- Easy for the nurse and patient to see each other and the screen.

Disadvantages
- Possible discomfort from the loss of a physical barrier between the nurse and patient
- Possible resistance to the increased prominence of the computer.

Over to you

For more detail and discussion of these arrangements go to:
www.gp-training.net/training/iicr/calcam.htm

Physical appearance

As with body posture, physical appearance provides information in an instant. It is one of the most immediate brief signals of our identity, status, role and our intentions. How we dress will be one of the first things that people notice and influences what their first impression of us will be. Professional uniforms are powerful signals to others about the expertise or expert knowledge of the wearer. While this may be reassuring in healthcare settings at one level, uniforms may also promote interpersonal distance.

In diverse health settings across hospital and community services, practitioners will need to take careful note of cultural expectations in terms of clothing. How we manage this key, brief communication may have far-reaching consequences for patients and clients. Wearing a uniform in Accident and Emergency may be reassuring to patients that they are being seen by experts, yet being identifiable as a health professional might provoke anxiety among mental health clients receiving a home visit due to the potential for being stigmatised in their community.

Touch

As with other communication strategies, such as direct eye contact or smiling, touch is an important means of building a relationship with other people. Whether we touch people, and how we do this, brings yet more dynamics to communication.

Our experience of touch throughout the lifespan will have an impact on our physiological, psychological and social wellbeing. For example, touch stimulation can increase interaction and weight gain in pre-term and newborn babies (e.g. Field *et al.* 2004), reduces aggression in infants and adolescents (Field 1999a, 1999b) or as Hernandez-Reif *et al.* (1999) found can even reduce smoking cravings.

So whether other people are touching us, we are touching them or even ourselves, there appear to be real benefits to our well being. This has been further established in research into the benefits of massage therapy in a wide range of physical and psychological health problems, such as anorexia (e.g. Hart *et al.* 2001) or asthma (Field *et al.* 1998). Yet we know that people in hospital may not always receive the touch they require. For example, Hollinger and Buschmann (1993) found that older adults in hospital received less tactile contact and Routasalo's (1999) literature review identified that male nurses touch less and male patients are touched less. Given the evidence for the benefits of touch, practitioners should look to employ this activity in an appropriate, culturally sensitive way.

Yet touch is a more skilled intervention than you would at first imagine (Bonham 2004). Some of the issues for the thoughtful nurse are about the places where you can touch a patient when you are nursing them. What difference does it make if your patient is male or female, 4 or 14 or 94 years old? A conservative and probably very safe approach is to never touch patients unless it is during the process of 'intimate nursing' such as helping people go to the toilet or bathing or eating, and so on. If you are going to touch patients in your communications, stick to the most legitimate sites: hands, arms, shoulders.

The limits and degree of what is appropriate quickly becomes apparent depending on the patient's needs, abilities and deficits. For example, the mildly confused 80-year-old women may need a different level of touch contact, compared to the semi-conscious young victim of a road accident. It is often quite easy to tell when your attempts to use touch as a helping medium are inappropriate as the patient will somehow tell you. They may not even use words. You will just sense a discomfort that tells you to alter your strategy.

If in doubt, keep touch to a minimum in anything other than the intimate nursing scenarios illustrated above. An example of touch perhaps being appropriate could be if someone is in a state of emotional upset (not necessarily a patient – it could be a relative or even a colleague). In this instance they may find a light touch on the hand, or shoulder or arm, very comforting. It is always advisable to ask permission first, unless you are very confident that you have the sort of relationship with the person that would make this kind of contact OK. On the other hand if you are trying to pacify someone who is angry, touching them may be misinterpreted as a threat or inflammatory gesture which could well escalate the situation that you are trying to calm. Just think of the times you have heard someone say 'Don't touch me!' when they are angry.

We must remember, of course, that people will have preferences in terms of how they communicate and how they expect others to communicate with them. The issue of how well attuned a health care professional is to the client's preferred means of communicating is important. If health care professionals make decisions or communicate in a way which fails to account for a client's cultural beliefs and preferences, then the client's self care, adherence to advice and overall outcome may well be poorer (Stewart *et al.* 1999).

As health practitioners we need to 'tune-in' to the communicating style and preferences of others in order to enhance care delivery. For example, if touch is used in communication with someone who is clearly indicating they are uncomfortable with this level of interaction, there may be all kinds of negative consequences. Equally, avoiding touch may convey rejection for others. The key thing is to strive to tailor our style of communicating with others rather than adopt a 'one-size-fits-all' approach.

Reflective activity

Think of an occasion where your touch seemed to help a person in your care. Why did it help? Think of an occasion where your touch didn't seem to help. Why didn't it help?

Top tips

As with the physical space you keep between yourself and patients, it is preferable and safer to be conservative about the way you use touch when you are nursing. Always ask permission before you touch a patient. If you are unsure then don't do it until you have checked with one of your colleagues who knows the patient well.

Reflective activity

Think of different styles of communication associated with different kinds of emotional tone. How would you speak and act if you were being:

- Bullied?
- Nervous?
- Confident?
- Humorous?
- Consider a recent example of your communication that did not seem to be acceptable to the other person
- What was the context of the communication, e.g. did it happen during a family visit, at the GP's, at the pub?
- How did the person object?
- How did this make you feel?
- What was your response? If this was unsatisfactory, what would you do next time?
- List examples of clinical situations in which you might need to make a careful assessment of preferred communication styles.

Relaxed manner

This is another paradoxical aspect of our professional communication rather like eye contact (see above) being most appropriate when it is not noticeable. Sometimes as a professional and effective nurse you will find that the situations that need you to be most relaxed are exactly the ones where you feel tense. For example, dealing with the family member who comes to visit their relative (your patient) on your hospital ward, and then seeks you out to complain about their treatment. If you are not expecting this (it's not happened before, usually the relative is quiet and uncomplaining, you are not aware of any difficulties with the patient) then it can be very shocking to be on the receiving end of a barrage of complaints that can feel very personal (as if you are personally responsible). The degree of relaxation needed here is a fine piece of nursing judgement. If you are tense and agitated, outwardly, the situation may well escalate out of your control, and as the professional here it is important that you retain control, without being over-controlling. If you are totally relaxed, or appear to be, the same result may be achieved; that is, you may well worsen the situation. You could appear to be uncaring, as not taking the matter seriously or accused of 'letting things lie'; that is, not dealing with the complaint.

Nursing is a job where the occasions when we are *totally* relaxed are few and far between. That is why the work is so tiring, even for nurses who work in clinical settings where the completion of tasks is not the prime objective of the job. You are constantly on alert. The skill is in you presenting yourself as being appropriately relaxed for the situation in which you find yourself, as a professional nurse.

Reflective activity

Here are some scenarios to illustrate a range of possibilities where being relaxed is important to optimise patient care but just as important is the degree of relaxation you show to the world. For each scenario answer the question: How relaxed would you appear?

1. *A patient is about to go to theatre for a surgical procedure. They want to go through with it but are clearly very frightened. You are thinking 'I'd hate to have that done'*

2. *A colleague, who is also your close friend, is about to go for an important interview. They are as nervous as you've ever seen them*

3. *A newly admitted patient has just collapsed right in front of you, on the ward. You kneel down beside them. They are an awful colour, and you can't immediately find a pulse. The student who is with you is starting to panic*

4. *A patient's father is visiting the ward. He smells strongly of alcohol and is starting to be verbally abusive to some of the other patients*

Key points

Core interpersonal skills involve:

- making yourself approachable and available to patients
- smiling, naming, welcoming and greeting them
- using ordinary, polite and dignified language
- appropriately using mutual gaze or eye contact, posture, body space (proximity) and touch
- maintaining a relaxed, appropriate outward appearance
- appropriately using praise and humour

Top tips

Create warmer communication by:

- smiling more
- using mutual gaze
- using appropriate touch to comfort, relax, show positive regard of individuals
- mirroring the posture of the patient or client where possible
- being willing to use all media to connect with others
- using positive, friendly gestures

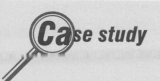

Case study

Ruth works as a midwife in a busy antenatal clinic in a large teaching hospital. She interviews mothers-to-be in her small office. Since Ruth has to deal with a high number of consultations each day she makes them businesslike and short in duration. The door to the office is always left half open and when mothers enter Ruth is usually facing away from them, staring at the computer terminal and entering information via the keyboard. Without looking around she says 'Take a seat' and proceeds to ask a series of questions, typing each answer into the electronic file.

● How would you feel if you were the mother?

● In what ways might Ruth's communication style affect the kinds of information that the mother-to-be shares with her?

● How would you do things differently?

RRRRRRapid recap

Check your progress so far by working through each of the following questions.

1. What can a higher pitch of voice convey?
2. What promotes attraction or likeability; indicates attentive listening and encourages disclosure?
3. What is the formal term for 'chit chat' or 'small talk'?
4. What do you call the exchange, return or reciprocation of eye contact?
5. What does the acronym SOLER stand for?

If you have difficulty with more than one of the questions, read through the section again to refresh your understanding before moving on.

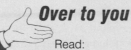

Over to you

Read:
Bonham, P. (2004) *Communicating as a Mental Health Carer.* Nelson Thornes, Cheltenham.

References

Adler, R., and Towne, N. (1999) *Looking Out, Looking In*, 9th edn. Forthworth, Harcourt Brace.

Argyle, M. (1994) *The Psychology of Interpersonal Behaviour.* Penguin, London.

Bonham, P. (2004) *Communicating as a Mental Health Carer.* Nelson Thornes, Cheltenham.

Brown, P. and Levinson, S. (1987) *Politeness: Some universals in language usage.* Cambridge University Press, Cambridge.

Brown, C. and Sulzerazaroff, B. (1994) An assessment of the relationship between customer satisfaction and service friendliness. *Journal of Organizational Behavior Management,* **14**, 55–75.

Burnard, P. (2003) Ordinary chat and therapeutic conversation: Phatic communication and mental health nursing. *Journal of Psychiatric and Mental Health Nursing,* **10**(6), 678–682.

Clements, P.T., Benasutti, K.M. and Henry, G.C. (2001) Drawing from experience: Using drawings to facilitate communication and understanding with children exposed to sudden traumatic deaths. *Journal of Psychosocial Nursing and Mental Health Services*, **39**(12), 12–20.

Davis, S. F. and Pallidino, J.J. (2000) *Psychology*, 3rd edn. Prentice-Hall, Upper Saddle River, NJ.

Duggan, A. and Parrott, R. (2001) Physicians' non-verbal rapport building and patients' talk about the subjective component of illness. *Human Communication Research,* **27**, 299–311.

Field, T. (1999a) Preschoolers in America are touched less and are more aggressive than preschoolers in France. *Early Child Development and Care*, **151**, 11–17.

Field, T. (1999b). American adolescents touch each other less and are more aggressive toward their peers as compared with French adolescents. *Adolescence*, **34**, 753–758.

Field, T., Henteleff, T., Hernandez-Reif M., Martinez, E., Mavunda, K., Kuhn C. and Schanberg, S. (1998). Children with asthma have improved pulmonary functions after massage therapy. *Journal of Pediatrics*, **132**, 854–858.

Field, T., Hernandez-Reif, M and Freedman, J. (2004). Stimulation programs for preterm infants. *Social Policy Report*, **18**, 1–19.

Hargie, O., Dickson, D. and Tourish, D. (1999) *Communication in Management*. Gower, Aldershot.

Hart, S., Field, T. Hernandez-Reif, M., Nearing, G., Shaw, S., Schanberg, S. and Kuhn, C. (2001). Anorexia symptoms are reduced by massage therapy, *Eating Disorders*, **9**, 289–299.

Hernandez-Reif, M., Field, T. and Hart, S. (1999). Smoking cravings are reduced by self-massage. *Preventive Medicine*, **28**, 28–32.

Holli, B. and Calabrese, R. (1998) *Communication and Education Skills for Dietetics Professionals*. 3rd edn. Williams & Wilkins, Baltimore.

Hollinger, L. and Buschmann, M. (1993) Factors influencing the perception of touch by elderly nursing home residents and their health caregivers. *International Journal of Nursing Studies* **30**, 445–61.

Kurtz, S., Silverman, J., Benson, J. and Draper, J. (2003) Marrying content and process in clinical method teaching: Enhancing the Calgary-Cambridge Guides. *Academic Medicine* **78**(8), 802–809.

Kurtz, S.M., Silverman, J.D. and Draper, J. (1998) *Teaching and Learning Communication Skills in Medicine*. Radcliffe Medical Press, Oxford.

LaFrance. M. and Hecht, M. (1999) Option or obligation to smile: the effects of power and gender on facial expression. In: *The Social Context of Non-verbal Behavior* (eds Philippot, P., Feldman, R. and Coats, E.) Cambridge University Press, Cambridge.

Malinowski, B. (1922) *Argonauts of the Western Pacific: An account of native enterprise and adventure in the archipelago of Melanesian New Guinea*. Routledge, London.

Martin R.A. (2001) Humor, laughter, and physical health: Methodological Issues and Research Findings. *Psychological* Bulletin, **127**(4), 504–519.

Monahan, J. (1998) I don't know it but I like you: The influence of nonconscious affect on person perception. *Human Communication Research*, **28**, 298–312.

Rao, P.R. (1995) Drawing and gesture as communication options in a person with severe aphasia. *Topics in Stroke Rehabilitation*, **2**(1), 49–56.

Rosenfeld, H. and Hancks, M. (1980) The non-verbal context of verbal listener responses. In *The Relationship of Verbal and Non-verbal Communication* (ed. Kay, M.) The Hague: Mouton.

Routasalo, P. (1999) Physical touch in nursing studies: A literature review. *Journal of Advanced Nursing*, **30**, 843–50.

Silverman, J.D., Kurtz, S.M. and Draper, J. (1998) *Skills for Communicating with Patients*. Radcliffe Medical Press, Oxford.

Stewart, A.L., Napoles-Springer, A. and Perez-Stable, E. (1999) Interpersonal processes of care in diverse populations. *Millbank Quarterly*, **77**(3), 305–339.

Wellings, T. (2001) Drawings by dying and bereaved children. *Paediatric Nursing* **13**(4), 30–31.

3 Critical reflection, assessment and basic counselling skills

Learning outcomes

By the end of this chapter you should be able to:

- Understand the need for reflection in communication
- Describe skills involved in assessment
- Identify models, frameworks or approaches for basic counselling
- Describe how rapport or a therapeutic relationship can be developed with others
- Understand the importance, use and value of basic counselling skills

Introduction

Nurses communicate in day-to-day spoken and written interactions with other members of the health care team, and patients and relatives. In the course of their work they will engage in all kinds of communication, not least assessments and interviews, where the right questioning technique can prove vital. The nurse will seek to build a therapeutic relationship with patients – sometimes within very limited time frames – and engage in some level of counselling. Each of these areas in care delivery will be explored further. In doing so, it will be evident that the way in which nurses use language, and reflect on their use of words and phrases, contributes either positively or negatively to the care provided.

Reflection and communication

We know that language enables you to describe and potentially transform nursing care, and that reflecting on this activity will promote professional awareness and growth. For nursing to achieve these ends, it must regularly and vigorously examine its practices and the values that underpin them, and the public's expectations of nurses and nursing care. Where there is no examination of practice and underlying theory, a profession stagnates.

The reflective approach demands that every aspect of the individual's nursing practice should be subjected to critical scrutiny in order to justify the care being provided. It is through such rigorous inquiry that nurses increase their awareness of and insight into the values, beliefs and motives of patients, clients and carers and are ultimately able to offer a service which is tailored to the unique needs of individuals rather than to the presumed needs of groups. This approach, championed by Schön (1983), is based on the belief that people can actually effect change through the raising of consciousness about what they do. This is something that needs to occur in terms of how we communicate with others and the language we use to do this.

Brykczynska (1995) argues that reflective practice is a means of thinking about oneself in the world, the impact which the world has on the practitioner and the impact that the practitioner has on the world. To be able to be truly reflective practitioners, she argues, nurses need to make a huge leap forward in the way they think about and act in their professional roles. Reflective practice requires nurses to question the way in which they deliver care, the knowledge which underpins it and the power relationships which drive it. They are required to ask hard questions such as: 'What do I know?', 'How do I know it?', 'Is it the best knowledge available?', 'Have I evidence to support what I am doing?'.

The quality of care will only improve as nurses (and other health professionals) develop critical reflection about how they communicate. For example, a nurse describes a particular piece of interaction in the following terms:

> I said something like "How are you doing Paul?" When he predictably answered "fine" I could easily have gone out the door and on with my work, but just by the way he answered I could tell he had much more to say. I asked Paul if he would like me to stay awhile and he replied that he would . . . For almost an hour I just listened to Paul as he talked about his life, his achievements, the risks he had and hadn't taken and his hopes for his limited future . . . When I stood up to go, his eyes met mine and we thanked each other in silence.
>
> (Perry 1996, p. 9)

This extract shows a number of important things about the caring work of nurses. Aside from meeting the patient's physical needs the nurse tuned in to Paul's desire for company and companionship. Furthermore, she probed beyond the patient's assertion that he is 'fine' – to create an experience that is rewarding to both nurse and patient. This example highlights the importance of being aware of the value of communication in enhancing the quality of life of patients. Of course, often nurses will not be able to allocate the extended block of time for this kind of communication offered to Paul. But nurses should strive to give as much time as possible to empathic communication and interaction within the real world of busy health settings. At the very least, this may be done in and around completing a variety of other nursing tasks.

In recognising the impact of humane communication with patients, nurses are in a key position to promote and influence the language and communication environments in which health care takes place. This role should extend to spoken, written and non-verbal communication and includes taking appropriate action if patients are subjected to negative, damaging interactions. This critical listening, observation and reading of communication does not simply mean that nurses should monitor their own performance, but importantly, that of other health care professionals. Yet nurses will only gain the right and indeed the skills to challenge the communication of others, by first reflecting critically on how they interact verbally and non-verbally themselves.

If we are to take the challenge of reflective practice seriously, this will involve addressing nursing on a number of fronts. Nurses need to become increasingly aware of the way that values are transmitted in spoken and written language and that nursing as a profession is constantly being described and positioned in particular ways by policy makers, health care managers etc. They need to examine more critically the way that they are being described and whether these descriptions of what they are and do support or undermine the core values of nursing. Reflective practice then, at its best, can enable nurses to understand the controlling influence of language. Without this reflective ability nursing can become the instrument of politically driven health agendas, which promote a task-focused service, or a factory-style processing of people, which may be far from the caring, compassionate approach it has always prided itself on. With this in mind, let us now move on to explore the key area of interviewing and assessing patients and clients.

Key points ~~Top tips~~

- How nurses use language, and reflect on their use of words and phrases, contributes either positively or negatively to the care provided
- Language enables you to describe and potentially transform nursing care and reflecting on this activity will promote professional awareness and growth
- Nurses are in a key position to promote and influence the language and communication environments in which health care takes place
- Reflective practice at its best can enable nurses to understand the controlling influence of language

Assessment

Assessment by interviewing is a core activity in health care, carried out in a variety of clinical environments or in people's homes. Often, this activity is conducted as part of care delivered by a number of health professionals working together to ensure a quality seamless service for the patient between home and health or social care institutions.

Assessment, even with very vulnerable or frail older adults should include the client as an active collaborator in the assessment process, be the basis for care plans that help users achieve their personal goals (Department of Health 1998), and adopt a multidisciplinary approach, especially where an individual has complex needs (Department of Health 1997).

Assessment process

The process of assessment can be an exhausting and frustrating experience for service users and carers, not least when they have to repeat their stories to several different health professionals conducting specific assessments using a variety of questionnaires and interview schedules peculiar to different professional groups (Health Committee 1999). However, there are increasingly more examples of interagency patient-held records so as to maximise not only the availability of a range of information to interested professionals, but also give the client a greater sense of ownership over their plan of care (Dunstan 1999). Nolan and Caldock (1996) make some suggestions for best practice in carrying out assessments (see p. 62).

As should be clear, all of these criteria are based on good communication and an acknowledgement of the central role of the client's perspective in the assessment process.

Models, frameworks or approaches in counselling

There are various theoretical models, frameworks or approaches available to guide nurse counselling and analyse communication approaches (see Box 3.2). These can be investigated as part of a nurse's commitment to continuing professional development and portfolio keeping.

Box 3.2: Key models or frameworks

1. Interpersonal Relations Model (Hildegard Peplau)
2. Client-Centred Therapy (Carl Rogers)
3. The Skilled Helper (Gerard Egan)
4. Six-Category Intervention Analysis (John Heron)
5. Transactional Analysis (Eric Berne)

Other Related Models, Frameworks or Approaches

1. Solution Focused Therapy (Steve De Shazer)
2. Emotional Intelligence (Antonio R. Damasio/various writers)
3. The JO-HARI Window (Joseph Luft and Harry Ingham)

You may, for example, want to start by looking at Peplau's Interpersonal Relations model, with its four phases: orientation, identification, exploitation and resolution (see Box 3.3) and six nursing roles (see Box 3.4).

Box 3.3: Peplau's four phases to interpersonal relations

1. *Orientation* – the client and nurse meet for the first time and there is a need to develop trust and empower the client
2. *Identification* – together the client and nurse identify problems that need to be worked on in the relationship
3. *Exploitation* – the client uses available services offered
4. *Resolution* – when all the client's needs are met, he/she becomes independent once more, and the current relationship with the nurse is closed

Over to you

Read from:

Simpson, H. (1991) *Peplau's Model in Action*. Palgrave Macmillan, Basingstoke.

Peplau, H.E. and Simpson, H. (1994) *Selected Works: Interpersonal Theory in Nursing*. Palgrave Macmillan, Basingstoke.

Box 3.4: Peplau's six nursing roles

1. *Counselor* – working with the patient on their problems
2. *Leader* – promoting a democratic relationship with the patient
3. *Surrogate* – standing in for a person in the patient's life
4. *Stranger* – accepting the patient as a new and unknown phenomenon
5. *Resource* – interpreting care plans for the patient
6. *Teacher* – providing information and facilitating learning

You may also wish to look at Heron's (1990) six category intervention, where he identifies two sets of interventions: those that are authoritative or nurse-directed (prescriptive, informative, confronting) and those that are facilitative or enable patients to develop themselves in some way (cathartic, catalytic, supporting) (see Box 3.5).

Box 3.5: Heron's (1990) six category intervention analysis

1. *Prescriptive* – directing, delegating, advising
2. *Informative* – factually informing, explaining
3. *Confronting* – challenging patient perspectives, attitudes or behaviour
4. *Cathartic* – encouraging expression of emotions
5. *Catalytic* – promoting further self-discovery
6. *Supportive* – valuing, accepting

This framework and others like it can help nurses reflect on and shape the kind of work they are doing when counselling and communicating with patients.

○━┳ *Keywords*

Rapport
Useful or harmonious relationship

Rapport and the therapeutic relationship

The **rapport** we have with patients is an indication of the quality of our relationship with them (Silverman, *et al*. 2005). A constructive or positive rapport is the first indicator that we are going to be able to help that patient although it may not be clear exactly how.

Some of the signs of a positive rapport can be as follows:

1. The communication (not necessarily verbal!) is two-way and balanced.
2. It is given and received with honesty and directness.
3. There is a sense of consistency and continuity, even through difficult patches.

The rapport that we have with patients we nurse is a unique function of the way we are with them, and the way they are with us. It is the nurse who is responsible for creating or leading the quality of the rapport. The patient will react to that lead. With a constructive rapport between a nurse and a patient, the nurse is more able to carry out the job of nursing in an effective, efficient, **holistic** and humane way.

As this is probably what most patients would like for themselves, it is the nurse's role to 'tune in' as the rapport develops. In very general terms you will see that some nurses seem to generate a very relaxed, almost informal, rapport with patients, while others are more formal and businesslike in their approach. Again this can be influenced by the context or setting in which the nurse is working. There can be very sound reasons why nurses present themselves in a particular way to a patient group.

In some situations the rapport may need extra energy to sustain it. When times get difficult the strength and depth of the rapport will be tested. Often, if sufficient investment has been made in the relationship, it will survive the hard times and may even be strengthened by them. For example as a nurse, you may be the 'messenger' required to ask the patient to comply with a treatment programme that is very likely to make them feel worse before they feel better. Here, as always, the emphasis is on asking negotiation and reaching an agreement that this is the best course of action. Reaching an agreement or **concord** will be more likely if you have worked hard to establish a trusting relationship with the individual.

Some cancer treatments may fall into this category. Or, in mental health settings you might be telling a patient that they are unable to go home because of the section of the Mental Health Act which detains them in hospital. You may be trying to persuade a young child to have medication via an injection, which you know will hurt them.

○━┳ *Keywords*

Holistic
All-enveloping or complete, taking all aspects of a person into account not just the illness

○━┳ *Keywords*

Concord/concordance
Negotiated agreement to pursue course of action – such as a treatment or medication

Reflective activity

Think about a patient you have a good rapport with, and one that you struggle to relate to.

What are the differences between the two patients?

How are you different when you are with them?

Remember, developing a therapeutic relationship with patients or clients requires courteous communication from the start. Without courtesy such a relationship is impossible – and we should not take it for granted that we use courteous language. Rather, we should be prepared to reflect critically on how we talk to others, whether in terms of how we meet and greet patients or refer to them in formal or informal ways, or the way we position our bodies as discussed in terms of SOLER in the previous chapter.

> ### Top tips
>
> You can start to work on your rapport with patients from the moment you first meet them. This is an essential precursor to the therapeutic relationship that might follow.

Warmth (being warm)

A key ingredient in gaining rapport with patients will be demonstrating that you are a 'warm' individual. It may help to understand more fully the idea of 'warmth' and what it feels like, if we first look at the idea of being 'cold' in our relationships with patients. Imagine that you are admitting, and therefore perhaps meeting, a patient for the first time. What are the feelings the patient may get if you greet them with a 'cool' or cold demeanour? They may feel rejected or not accepted, despondent, perhaps judged, even aggressive. Given the situation you are in, as the professional, any therapeutic process that was going to be possible (this applies to any nursing clinical situation), will now be so much more difficult.

To get a sense of how 'warmth' might alter the above situation, just substitute the *opposite* meanings for all the above descriptions. We now have: accepted, optimistic or hopeful, treated in a non-judgemental way, peaceful (or at least not aggressive). The way that you model warmth is similar to the way you model approachability. An open, friendly, respectful demeanour, together with the offer of comforting gestures such as somewhere to sit down, or a drink (if appropriate to the circumstances) all help create that all-important first impression.

Attempting to be empathic (empathising)

At the heart of gaining a patient's trust and creating a therapeutic relationship, is empathy – that is, attempting to enter into and show that you understand something of what it might be like being that person, in particular circumstances, in conversation with you or communication through non-verbal channels. This requires imagination on your part – as we cannot enter into the minds of others – but showing empathy will result from a thoughtful consideration of the information that another person provides or that you can glean from observation of their situation and the challenges they face. As we noted in the previous chapter, how we position our bodies in relation to others will signal empathy. Or indeed, we show it by the warmth of our response to them, perhaps through a sympathetic smile or touch.

Some of the ways of explaining this concept are ideas such as: 'Standing in the other person's shoes' or 'Seeing the world through the other person's eyes' or 'Having a sense of what the other person has experienced or is experiencing'.

It is *not* being in the position of being able to say to a patient 'I know how you feel'. If you look at life events such as giving birth, losing a loved relative, getting divorced, being in a road accident, being overdrawn at the bank, having an argument with your neighbour, many of us have a sense of what that is like, or what it *may* be like. However, we cannot know *exactly* what it is like for another person to go through that experience. But often, the nurse can offer a useful contribution to the **intervention** they have with a patient, even in very difficult circumstances.

In terms of counselling, we also convey empathy by accurately reflecting and summarising people's feelings, completing a 'feedback loop' which returns the message to the patient that you are *attempting* to enter into their 'world-view'. In the example below the patient has been given a piece of very difficult news by a doctor. As is often the case, the news has now sunk in, and some of the repercussions start to raise questions that the patient tries to clarify with the nurse:

Derek: Nurse, excuse me a minute. The doctor I saw this morning said that it would be best for me to have that operation. I've been thinking. I really don't want to have it. I can't bear the thought of living like that.

Nurse: You look really shaken.

Derek: You're absolutely right. I hadn't realised what I signed up for. John over there has just had the same thing and look at the state of *him* now.

Nurse: You sound terrified.

Derek: I bloody am!

You can track the course of this conversation easily. The nurse is making accurate empathic interventions. You can tell that they are accurate because of the response from the patient. Here, the patient

Keywords

Intervention
Any contact of any kind that you have with a patient. The term does not necessarily indicate that a verbal exchange needs to happen

is revealing very quickly his hidden fears (within three sentences). This is making things more difficult for the nurse as she is getting into a very tricky situation in terms of the quality and thoughtfulness of her responses to Derek's distress. However, had she not made the empathic attempt in the first place, Derek may not have been presented with a safe opportunity to voice his concerns.

Reflective activity

Now that you have some understanding of what being empathic means, try to recall an occasion when you were, at least in some way, empathic with another person at work (not necessarily a patient).

What were the circumstances?

What did you say to the person in your attempt to be empathic?

How did they respond to you to confirm that you were being empathic?

How helpful was this to you in your role as a nurse?

How helpful was this to the other person?

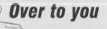

Over to you

Try to construct empathic interventions when you are in conversation with another person, not just in work situations. Try to imagine how they must feel about the situation that they are in, and say something that shows you have some inkling of how they are at that moment. Don't be put off if your attempts seem clumsy at first. You are likely to find that in many instances the other person will appreciate that you are making the attempt to understand in some way.

Active listening and attending

As the term implies, when you are doing this, you are carrying out an activity. That activity is difficult to do. It sometimes seems to take a lot of energy and thoughtful persistence. That is why the active listener can feel so tired after long periods of active listening.

It is important to remember that people often require clear signals that you are actively listening to them. It is therefore necessary to use an appropriate level of verbal prompts such as 'yes', 'mmm', 'go on', 'I see', 'how interesting' or 'OK' and non-verbal prompts such as nodding, smiling, etc. Also, avoid fiddling with objects while conversing, or looking away or over the patient's shoulder – 'shoulder surfing'. Just remember how this feels when it happens to you! With care, you should be able to convey that you are interested in what the person is saying and really attend to them. By actively listening in a genuine way to what patients have to say (rather than thinking about what you are going to say next), or simply giving time to share your 'presence' with them, you will begin the process of gaining rapport or bonding with the patient. You can do this by saying almost nothing but just maintaining steady eye contact as the person is speaking and occasionally nodding your head as if to say 'Yes, go on' or 'I see' (Burnard 1992).

Asking appropriate questions at appropriate times

There are different forms of questions that can be used in basic counselling and communicating with clients. There are two main kinds of questions: open and closed. Open questions do not result in 'yes' and 'no' answers as in closed questions, where answers will be a matter of straightforward fact, as witnessed in admissions: e.g. 'Do you have any allergies?'. Open questions facilitate a greater exploration of ideas and exchange of information. For example, if you ask a person, 'Are you in pain?' the answer would usually be a bald 'yes' or 'no'. However, if you asked 'What is the pain like?' you would normally receive a longer account or response.

Many books on the subject of interpersonal skills suggest that the use of open questions – What? Where? How? Who? Why? – will cause people to 'open up' to you. There is widespread agreement that patient-centred communication, which uses open questions, and tries to elicit the patient's full range of concerns and problems,

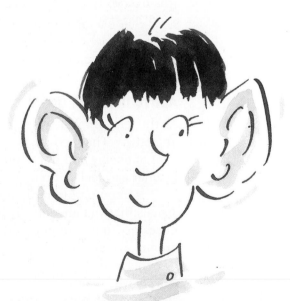

I'm all ears.

improves patient's health status and increases the efficiency of care (Chan *et al.* 2003, Stewart *et al.* 2000). That said, it is best to avoid questions beginning with 'why' because this tends to suggest that judgement is being passed on what a patient has, or has not done.

Another form of questioning is 'ranking', where a patient is asked to place items in order of importance. This can be useful, for example, when trying to decide which problems the patient feels need to be prioritised.

An important part of the skill of basic counselling is to hold back from asking too many questions. This is a common mistake made by less experienced nurses who are just discovering how to use 'open questions' and can close down the interaction rather than encourage it, attracting 'I don't know' as a response to their probing.

Reflective activity

Think how you might feel when confronted by a nurse, who you've just met, who seems to need to know things about you that very few other people know and begins firing a series of questions. How do you respond under the pressure of multiple questions?

Questions need to be posed selectively and carefully. The nurse will need to consider issues of privacy, and frame any questions to avoid: (a) seeming intrusive, particularly where topics are sensitive, for example in relation to sexual health, or other potentially embarrassing areas of care; (b) making the patient uncomfortable, particularly where rapport has not been fully established or developed; (c) adding to stress and frustration resulting from any communication difficulties, confusion or anxiety; (d) appearing cold or lacking emotional warmth; (e) coming across as rude or impolite.

On some admission paperwork you may find questions like 'What is the patient's understanding of their illness?' You will see that the nature of this question is very different from that of the earlier admission questions above. There are some things that the professional nurse needs to take into account before asking these questions, so that the admission can be carried out in the most efficient, yet the most caring way, possible.

Consider first the possibilities of asking this type of question exactly as it is presented on the admission form. Here are some examples of what might happen:

Nurse: What is your understanding of your illness?
Patient 1: I don't bloody know – you're the nurse!

Patient 2: I've no idea. The GP said I needed to come into hospital as an emergency. I can't remember what she said.

Patient 3: It's not looking good is it?

Patient 4: I've looked on the internet, and what that doctor said to me is wrong.

So open questions can generate diverse responses from patients (and relatives and colleagues) that are sometimes difficult to answer. You can see from the examples above that straightaway the nurse has been put into a situation where she will have to be very skilled when giving a considered response.

As noted above, an aspect of the 'open question' that needs care on the part of the nurse is its ability to become part of an uncomfortable style of intervention for the patient:

Nurse: Morning, Gerald. Did you get a better night's sleep?

Gerald: Yes, not too bad – considering.

Nurse: Considering what?

Gerald: Well, you know, my head was spinning again.

Nurse: What do you mean?

Gerald: The thoughts. I can't seem to clear them.

Nurse: What thoughts are they?

Gerald: Just worries. You know . . .

Nurse: Go on.

Gerald: Oh I don't know . . .

Nurse: You must know.

Gerald: I can't talk about it right now.

So here is a series of open questions asked by the nurse that don't really lead anywhere and in fact seem to close things down in terms of Gerald being able to express his worries. Here the whole business of timing can be significant (Bonham 2004). The same, or similar, questions asked at a different time can work differently.

Later the same day:

Nurse: How's it going, Gerald?

Gerald: Fine thanks.

Nurse: I hope you have a better night than last night.

Gerald: Yes, maybe I'll be even more tired and perhaps sleep better.

Nurse: So what was worrying you again last night? I know you didn't want to say earlier.

Gerald: Yes, I know. I just felt a bit despondent about it all.

Nurse: Despondent about what?

Gerald: Well, I don't seem to be making any progress do I? It seems like two steps forward and three back.

Nurse: What do you see as the forward steps, Gerald?

The style of questioning isn't any different. The nurse focuses on the same concerns. He acknowledges Gerald's discomfort from earlier in the day, but this doesn't stop him gently challenging Gerald to try to find out a little more about how he really is.

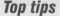

Reflective activity

Think of occasions when open questions have been helpful and effective for you, in terms of helping you help a patient, relative or colleague. Now think of occasions when their use has not helped, or has even made it more difficult. What made that difference?

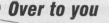

Top tips

Be careful and thoughtful about when and how you ask questions. It may be worth even trying to reduce the number of questions with which you bombard the patient.

Over to you

Try finding out about people by only asking questions sparingly, if at all. Listen instead and observe them more.

Responding to questions

It is important that nurses respond to questions in an honest and clear manner. You may think at first sight that this is relatively straightforward to do. You just tell 'the truth' in a direct manner. Consider the following example. A patient is worried about a surgical procedure they are about to undergo:

Doris: I'm really not looking forward to this. Do you think everything will be OK? I'm terrified I'll wake up from the anaesthetic during the operation. I saw a programme on the TV about it.

Nurse: I know. I saw it as well. The thought's really scary isn't it? I wouldn't fancy having an op either.

So here the nurse has just been honest and straightforward – but what is the impact of this honesty and directness on the patient? This skill of responding to questions from the recipients of our care

4. The impact of a statement can be truly experienced, e.g. 'I think you are working far too hard, and I'm very worried.' (Followed by a silence.)

> ☝ ***Over to you***
>
> In your conversations with people (not necessarily at work), try using periods of silence. See what the effect of this is. A good way to try this out is to allow a period of about four or five seconds to elapse after someone has finished speaking to you, before you start to talk. See how many times the other person adds something to what they have just said. You will find that in professional nursing settings, the 'add ons' are sometimes very important.

Clarifying

Clarifying is an essential basic skill that can make a big difference to the quality of your interactions with patients. It simply means making sure (as sure as you can be) that you really *do* understand what the patient is saying to you, in the fullest sense possible, at that moment. You can imagine that this has important implications for nurses who work with patients from different social, cultural and ethnic backgrounds who may speak the same language or communicate in a different language or in a **dialect** unfamiliar to us. Sometimes the situations that people are in appear fairly straightforward and at other times much more complex where checking out the meaning of what people say can be very important. Let us look at these in turn, starting with some fairly simple cases or issues. Here is an example of a nurse who is using the skill of clarifying to help the patient:

Tom: I want to go home. I'm fed up with this bloody place. It's making me worse.
Nurse: What do you mean *worse*, Tom?
Tom: I'm just left alone, all day.
Nurse: We're seeing you regularly through every shift, aren't we?
Tom: Yeah. I didn't mean you lot. You're doing your best, I suppose.
Nurse: So what are you getting at? What are you fed up about?
Tom: Where's Margaret and the lads? They never visit. They've forgotten I exist.
Nurse: What do you think about me nipping to get the phone for you, Tom? You can ring your wife then.

Here's another example of the nurse using clarifying skills:

Dawn: I've spoken to my mum. She says she doesn't want me to have anything to do with Darren. She reckons it's his fault I'm in this mess.

○━ᴛ *Keywords*

Dialect
A form of speech that occurs within a particular geographical area or region

Nurse: Nothing at all?
Dawn: Yeah.
Nurse: What about after the operation?
Dawn: I don't know. I'm not sure how I feel.
Nurse: About the operation, or not seeing Darren?
Dawn: No, about mum. I'm frightened what she might do to him if they meet again.

And another:

Nurse: Morning, Florence. Sleep OK?
Florence: So, so. Not too bad I suppose.
Nurse: Sounds like maybe you had a rough night again?
Florence: Well, I was OK 'til about 3.30. I had one of those dreams again. I couldn't get back to sleep.
Nurse: That's a shame. What was the dream about this time?

You can see from these examples that the outcome of the conversation could at worst be quite different and at best delayed if the nurse had not made the effort to clarify what the patient meant. Ambivalence or uncertainty can be a strong cue for using the skill of clarification, as in the examples above with Florence and Dawn. Here the nurse 'teases out' what seems to be a leading worry for the patient at that time.

As indicated above, clarifying or checking out the meaning of what people say is especially important when dealing with complex issues. The very nature of nursing means that inevitably, at some point in your work, you will be drawn into the patient's and/or the relative's questions or anxieties about what is happening to them. If you are concerned about or take account of the 'bigger picture' as part of the way you and the team work with patients, then it is essential that you become involved in some of these complex issues. This however, can create its own difficulties for the nurse. Consider the following examples – some are relatively simple, some are more complex – but they are *all* complex to the patient:

Jane: Do you think if my husband rings to find out how I am, you could be as vague as possible? Don't tell him anything about me, will you?
Nurse: OK. You don't want us to say anything at all? I'll pass that on to the other staff, if that's what you want.
Jane: Well, you could say I'm fine – just leave it at that will you?
Nurse: You're fine? Yes, we can say that. If that's what you want. Would you mind if I asked the reason you don't want him to know anything? This is a pretty big operation you're having, isn't it. He'll know that.

Jane: He'll know that, and it's got nothing to do with him anymore!

Nurse: What do you mean Jane?

Jane: He's had another affair. I've had it with him. It's over.

Nurse: I didn't know. So, you want to cut off from him completely?

Jane: I don't want to see him ever again.

Nurse: What about calls from other people?

Jane: Yes, if my mum calls please tell her how I am. I don't want anyone else involved.

Nurse: What about people from your work, the ones that called last week?

Jane: No, just mum.

Nurse: OK, Jane. I'll make sure that's in your notes. You'll let one of us know if you change your mind about this won't you?

Jane: That's very unlikely.

You can see here that Jane is struggling with many issues that are probably not connected with the surgery she is about to undergo. The problems will still be there on the other side of her operation. But so will the nurses who may be in a position to help Jane as she starts to manage her life again. The nurses can help just by listening to what Jane wants and being clear about this – just as the nurse above has done. In this first example, all the nurse has done is to make sure that she is clear about what it is that Jane wants. She has been accepting (Rogers 2003) of this and has carried out Jane's wishes, regardless of what she personally feels is 'right'. The issue here is that Jane only wants information about her given to one other person. The story underneath this is complicated and painful for her. At this point, however, the nurse manages the immediate need of the patient. She does this by clarifying and checking by minimal and non-intrusive questioning (Bonham 2004). Any other attempt to offer 'counselling' may be mistimed, inappropriate and may agitate Jane even more.

Here is a second example:

Robert (age 8): I don't want that thing in my ear anymore, I don't like it.

Nurse: I'll be ever so quick. I just need to see if your ear is still poorly inside. You said it felt a bit better since you've been having that medicine?

Robert: Yes, so why do you have to look?

Nurse: To check how much better your ear is, and to see if we're giving you the right kind of medicine.

Robert: I'm all right. I don't like it.

Nurse: What's bothering you?

Robert: I told my sister about that thing you put in my ear.

Nurse: What did Emma say about it?
Robert: Nothing.
Nurse: Sounds like she must have said something – so what was it?
Robert: Don't know.
Nurse: Did she worry you?
Robert: She said if it touched my brain, I'd die.
Nurse: Well, no wonder you don't want it in your ear – I wouldn't if I thought that was going to happen to me. Just give me a minute and I'll show you a picture of what the inside of your ear looks like. You'll see that what Emma suggested can't possibly happen to you. Will you have a look at it with me?
Robert: Let me see it.

This is a particularly difficult situation because of the age of the patient and his understanding of what is happening. The nurse attempts to explain things to Robert at a level that he may best understand, but only once she has really appreciated the cause of his fear, which in its way is quite rational. She demonstrates a form of what could be described as empathy when she implies that she wouldn't want her ear inspected either, if death was a possible outcome! She tries to persuade Robert by showing him a picture of the inside of an ear to reassure him. The hidden complexity here is that Robert is not necessarily bothered by the discomfort of having a probe pushed into his ear. He fears the consequences of this – his possible death. Only if the nurse gets to this stage can she continue effectively, and fully, to help him.

Here is example three:

Nurse: Martin, here are your tablets for the next week. Have you collected your things from your room?
Martin: Yes, I've got everything I think.
Nurse: Have a good time. Look after yourself properly. Don't do anything I wouldn't do!
Martin: Yeah, see you in a week. Will you be here then?
Nurse: Probably, I can't remember what shifts I'm doing. Anyway there's always someone here that you know isn't there?
Martin: Yeah . . . It's just if things go wrong again. . . .
Nurse: Wrong again? What do you mean?
Martin: Well . . . I don't know.
Nurse: Go on. What's bothering you?
Martin: Last time I went out for a week, I started hearing the neighbours swearing at me again. I could hear them talking about me through the walls – everywhere I went.
Nurse: So you think it may all happen again
Martin: I'm pretty sure it will. Do I have to go back there?

Nurse: You seem really worried about this. You're on different medication now. You've been fine on the ward for the past few weeks, haven't you? What stopped you bringing this up with your doctor when we discussed this leave with you?

Martin: He thinks I'm a time waster. He's never really listened to me all along.

Nurse: So, you've never wanted to do this at all?

Martin: No.

Nurse: OK. Let's sit down and have a think about this.

In this example, the nurse has gradually clarified that Martin has a poor relationship with his psychiatrist. This is destabilising an important stage of his rehabilitation. At an early stage of this conversation the nurse has clarified big ideas like '. . . if things go wrong again'. This has led to the patient's imagined consequences of things going wrong and the realisation that the foundations of the therapeutic relationship with one of his most significant carers is not all that it should perhaps be. Again, you can see in this example that the story starts with a patient's hesitancy to go home. Clarification, checking and careful questioning on the part of the nurse reveals something much more serious. Let us now turn to two key activities related to clarifying: paraphrasing and summarising.

Paraphrasing and summarising

A key strategy for aiding reflection on the content of what others say to us is the use of paraphrasing. This is not merely repeating what the other person says – 'parrot-phrasing' – but involves restating in brief what a patient has told you. The aim of this is to: (a) clarify that you have heard them accurately and that you are paying attention to what they say; (b) give an opportunity for both you and the patient to reflect on what was said (the content); and (c) encourage further development of ideas or issues. You may reflect back or acknowledge the feeling or emotion that a patient expressed verbally and non-verbally during conversation. This can deepen the sense of empathy and may help the patient review areas in his/her life where there are problems or opportunities that need addressing.

In summarising the content of a conversation with a patient, you will be better able to draw together the key aspects of what was communicated. This can help to bring a shape to what may have been an unstructured discussion, and may lead to exploring possible solutions to problems. Once you have established rapport and trust with a patient, negotiating solutions can occur in a creative process of formulating new approaches or strategies in relation to patient care and where unhelpful thinking or behaviours adopted by patients can be challenged and reframed into a new, more helpful perspective.

Key points **Top tips**

Practise paraphrasing and summarising. You can do this outside your work setting as well. You'll find with short interventions there is little difference between the two techniques. Over longer interventions, see how the two intervention styles can help your nursing practice by sifting out issues that are more and less important to the patient.

⊶ᴛ *Keywords*

Congruent
Being the same outside as inside, i.e. thinking the same as you behave

Authentic
Genuine or reliable

Showing genuineness, being non-judgemental, being accepting

Showing genuineness is all about being **congruent**, honest, **authentic** or real (Bonham 2004). The sense of this is that, as a professional, you have no tension between the way you think and feel inside your head, and the way the outside world sees you. This is a very simple idea, but again, as with many of these concepts the nursing reality is sometimes very different. There are situations in nursing that you are likely to face that may be upsetting, frightening, funny, embarrassing, upsetting and so on.

In some of these situations it will be difficult to conceal your true feelings but often it is the professional course of action to do so. For example, you meet George on the ward. He is a newly admitted patient who you do not know. In the course of shift handover you hear that he has a long history of drinking heavily, together with assaults on his family, and even sometimes the family's pet dogs. It is highly unlikely that anyone in the nursing team would approve of that lifestyle. However, when face to face with George, the majority of nurses – as professionals – manage to contain and put on one side their immediate personal thoughts about his behaviour. You may suggest that this is not being genuine or honest or congruent. In these instances, the professional nurse aspires to be these things, but perhaps sometimes falls short. You will see that experienced professional nurses manages to contain their own personal feelings about some patients, almost as if those feelings are in a box outside their immediate work situation. We therefore attempt to be accepting.

Imagine another setting. You are helping a patient get out of bed in the morning as they are a little unsteady on their legs. You suddenly realise that you have their faeces on your clothes and shoes. It is the first time that this has ever happened to you. The person is now standing, ready to walk and completely unaware of what is going on in your mind. They need constant, steady, unflustered assistance. You can see the tension!

Refl*Reflective activity*

Imagine that you are in this situation or some equivalent nursing situation – something that you are really repelled by.

How will you handle this?

What can you do to prepare yourself for a difficult scenario like this?

Using simple activities to promote communication

Using simple activities, such as bed making, helping with meals, making a drink, washing, or mobilising, can help promote relationships with patients. As well as having the obvious benefits of helping you 'tune in' to the needs of the patient you are working with (regardless of their age or clinical setting) and extend the range of data you are able to amass in terms of their assessment, simple activities can provide huge opportunities for the creative nurse to enrich the quality of the relationship with the patient.

For example, just helping a patient make their bed gives you the opportunity to do several valuable things. You can talk directly with them about the reasons they are in the care setting, e.g. their illness/deficit/disorder, if this is helpful and appropriate. This might lead on to them expressing their own understanding of what is happening to them, how they see it, what they need in that situation, and so on. This can all happen while you are actually making the bed, so your focus is not the bed, it's the patient. You can discuss their plans for the future and so get a feel for their levels of motivation and the degree of dependence on the care system of which they are currently the recipient. As you work together, you can look around and see what is around the bed area. Is it tidy or dishevelled? Is there a sense of order or disorder? How does that relate to the patient in your care? Is it typical of how they are, or untypical? What might all this indicate to you and the rest of the care team?

You may find as part of this activity that it's sometimes helpful to tell the patient a little about yourself. This is often described as **self disclosure**.

An example could go like this:

Joanne: I never like making my bed. I don't bother at home, what's the point?

Nurse: I see what you mean. I suppose I like the feeling of tidiness when I get home after being at work.

o—ᴨ *Keywords*

Self disclosure

Saying something to a patient about yourself, with the intention of helping the patient

Joanne: I've never been tidy. My mum's house was always a tip and I suppose I've inherited that, just like everything else.

Nurse: What else do you mean?

You can see that the little bit of self disclosure has given the patient the opportunity to, in turn, disclose a little more about her own life.

Similarly, imagine you are helping an elderly man to mobilise. He is recovering from a hip replacement:

John: Ooh that's sore. I'm struggling a bit here.

Nurse: You're doing fine. Don't forget, it's only a few days since you had the new hip.

John: Yes, but I'm sick of sitting around. I'd be working on the allotment if I was home.

Nurse: I know what you mean. Gardens can get away from you this time of the year, can't they? I'm weeding mine every weekend at the moment.

John: That's what I mean. It's all right for you. I don't know how I'm going to manage when I get home.

Nurse: You're doing really well, John. You can't rush these things. Your neighbour Fred is coming in later. He's got an allotment next to yours hasn't he? What do think about asking him to keep an eye on it for you?

Again, a little self disclosure from the nurse has indicated that she has some understanding of John's worries. At the same time she is positive, encouraging and supportive. She also makes a *tentative* suggestion as to how John may start to address his worries. (Note that he may not necessarily wish to do what the nurse is suggesting. It might, however, encourage a problem-addressing approach on the part of the patient.)

Reflective activity

Think about the problems that patients tell you about.

What proportion of these problems can nurses really help with?

What could be the nurses' role with regard to problems that nurses cannot directly help with?

4 Negotiation, empowerment, feedback and information

Learning outcomes

By the end of this chapter you should be able to:

- Understand the meanings and some of the practical applications of terms like: concordance, empowerment, non-stigmatising language, constructive feedback
- Describe skills involved in information giving, teaching and promoting health
- Appreciate the need for accurate and appropriate records
- Describe the legal and ethical issues around record keeping in health care
- Describe the role of patient advocacy

Keywords

Negotiation
Discussing or conferring to reach agreement

Concordance
A harmonious agreement that is achieved through negotiation

Compliance
Act of simply complying or going along with whatever is proposed

Introduction

This chapter will build further on some of the basic skills explained in earlier parts of this book. You will see how to use some of these skills concerned with negotiation and empowerment in more difficult situations and in a more sophisticated way. Some of the examples that are used in this chapter show how nurses can respond to people (not only patients) who present a number of different clinical challenges.

Negotiating care

When considering the process of **negotiation** with service users there is an important distinction to make between **concordance** and **compliance**. In other parts of this book we have tried to address the area of empowering patients (Watkins 2001), that is, doing as much as we reasonably can to help patients be involved in their own care, and be part of their own decision-making care team. In this spirit, we use the more contemporary term 'concordance'. We try to inform the patient about what is happening. They are part of their own care process, therefore, any decision about their care and any course of action taken as a result of that care is with their encouragement and support and backing. They are concordant and empowered at the same time. The term 'compliance' has a more dated sense of patients going along with a treatment programme because they feel they have little or limited choice, and maybe could be considered as disempowered, in relative terms.

Given this sense of the patient being a more powerful and influential partner in the relationship between nurse and patient (NMC 2002), some of the dilemmas that may result from this equality are as follows:

1. The patient may want what we (the professional carers) think is not appropriate or 'best' for them. For example, the patient may wish to go home or be discharged from a clinical area before we feel they are ready

2. The patient may wish to stop taking prescribed medication, or may wish to have more, or different, medication from that which has been prescribed

3. They may want conditions surrounding their treatment to be different from those which are governed by local policy, e.g. they may wish to have a large group of family visitors or friends, or may like to eat or drink at times that don't fit into the usual routine of the clinical area

4. They may want to complain about the care they have, or haven't had.

You can see that in all the examples above, reaching a compromise or at least a situation in which both the patient and their carers are reasonably satisfied with the outcome can be difficult to attain. Consider the following examples.

Tom: Excuse me, nurse. I thought I said I didn't want these tablets anymore. They're making me feel sick all the time. I don't think they're helping me anyway.

Nurse: Well, the doctor has prescribed them, so you'd better take them. You'll probably feel better when you've adjusted to them a little more. Who did you ask about this anyway?

Tom: I mentioned it to the staff last night. She said she'd sort it out.

Nurse: Well, it's the first I've heard. I'll try to catch the doctor later on to review your script.

Here Tom is no better off in his situation, in any respect. The nurse is trying to gently pressurise him to be compliant and take his medication, even though he has said that it makes him feel ill. There is no feeling of teamwork or continuity of communication across shifts when the nurse says that she doesn't know about Tom's request. The remark that Tom may feel better when he has 'adjusted' isn't very convincing, and may be seen as avoidance by the nurse, who hasn't really listened Tom's concerns.

See how the response of the second nurse is more aligned with a 'spirit of concordance'.

Tom: Excuse me, nurse. I thought I said I didn't want these tablets anymore. They're making me feel sick all the time. I don't think they're helping me anyway.

Nurse: OK, I didn't realise they were making you feel like that. I'll contact the doctor to review your medication. I'll omit them for the moment until I've spoken to her on the phone. I'll let you know what she says. How long have you been feeling sick?

Tom: I told the nurse last night. It's ever since I was first given them, but it's not getting any better.

Nurse: OK. I missed that bit. I'll let the doctor know, Tom. Is there anything else that's bothering you about your tablets while I'm here?

Tom: No. If you can sort that out, it would be good, thanks.

Reflective activity

Think of other examples from your practice where the nurse has acted in a spirit of concordance. How was that achieved by the nurse? What was the outcome of that approach? Think of examples from your practice where negotiated agreement (and therefore concordance) has not seemed to be possible. What were the reasons?

Top tips

The best top tip in these situations is to really listen to the patient. You need to do this before even attempting to nurse patients in a spirit of concordance.

Key points

- Seek a harmonious agreement with patients (concordance) rather than insisting upon compliance with care interventions
- Listen to the concerns of patients about proposed care

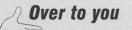

Over to you

When you are working with patients try to be aware of how you can achieve concordance rather than compliance. This is sometimes likely to be difficult. There is often pressure from other professionals to obtain compliance.

Empowering people

Keywords

Lateral (thinking)
An ability to think around a problem or create alternative ideas to try out

Using empowering language encourages self determination and decision making of others. It focuses around the needs and wants of the service user (Watkins 2001), requires creativity and **lateral thinking** (De Bono 1973), and a determined desire on the part of the nurse to help the patient to help themselves. Of course, doing this isn't easy.

Sometimes being disempowering seems like the easier course. Look at the two following examples in which the elderly patient, Jack, is about to go for his lunch at the day hospital he attends three times a week. He is sometimes a little confused:

Nurse: Jack, it's time for your dinner. Let's get you into the dining room. It's fish today. That's your favourite! Come on, it's getting cold.

It is clear that the nurse here is encouraging Jack to do what she thinks is appropriate, given the time of day and the occasion. There is nothing obviously wrong with the way that she gently cajoles him; after all, if he doesn't move he may miss his lunch or it might go cold, and there are other patients to see to, as well. Compare the first nurse's style with this:

Nurse: Hello, Jack. It's lunch time. Would you like to go through into the dining room to eat with the others? It's fish today – how do you fancy that? Do you want to go now with me? Or shall I come back for you in a few minutes?

You will notice straight away that the main difference between the two styles is that the second approach uses more questions and therefore implies more choice. The second interactional style is more focused around Jack's needs rather than the nurse's need to get things done.

Here is another example:

Mandy: I don't want to stay on this ward any longer. I'm not getting any better – it's making me worse. The other patients are all getting on my nerves.

Nurse: Yes, things have been a bit tricky this morning haven't they? Have you thought seriously about going? Do you want to go for the day or the weekend, or perhaps longer? We could sort something out with your doctor if you like? How about sticking with it a little longer? Things will probably be a little quieter now we've sorted out the new admission. Have a think anyway Mandy. Let me know what you decide then we can talk it through with Doctor Moss. I think she's around this afternoon.

Here, the nurse has responded to Mandy's concerns in an understanding way. She acknowledges that things have been difficult on the ward. She gives Mandy several options, including the consideration of staying. Also the nurse leaves the possibility of negotiation with the doctor open to Mandy.

Reflective activity

What might be causing Mandy to feel this way?

What other things might she want apart from her request to go?

What things might make it difficult for Mandy to go?

Nurse: Hilda, you're looking a bit lost today?

Hilda: I'm really worried about Jack. He's not had to look after himself for years. I've always done everything for him. I don't know how he'll manage without me.

Nurse: What do think he's going to struggle with?

Hilda: I don't know – everything I suppose.

Nurse: What do you think he'll need to get by, until you are home?

Hilda: I do all the shopping and cooking. He hasn't got a clue you know.

Nurse: Well, how is he managing now? Is there any food in the house?

Hilda: I did a big shop at the weekend, so yes he'll be OK for now, I suppose.

Nurse: So there's no immediate problem?

Hilda: No, but he can't manage you know.

Nurse: He's visiting tomorrow isn't he, after your tests? How about if we get together then? We could get our heads together and plan something to help him manage? You could think of some ideas to help him maybe, Hilda?

Hilda: Oh, OK. But he's still going to struggle – I know it.

Here the nurse is having difficulties reassuring Hilda who seems determined that her husband can't manage without her. Even if this is the case, the nurse has left a creative opportunity open for Hilda to stay engaged with sorting out the problems, rather than just ruminating about them.

elteR*Reflective activity*

How else might the nurse have managed the situation presented above?
What could be behind Hilda's anxieties?

Here is a fourth example:

Joan: I've been thinking of what the doctor said about that medication and the long-term effects it could have on me. He went through it all very carefully, but I've decided that I don't want to have it after all. I bet he'll be really fed up with me.

Nurse: I doubt that. He would have gone through all that stuff so that you could make a decision, even though he may disagree with you.

Joan: What do you think? Do you think I'm wrong as well?

Nurse: I didn't say you were wrong. It's your decision really. These drugs can have difficult side effects and it's the doctor's job, and ours sometimes, to make all this as clear as possible to you.

Joan: OK, but what do you think I should do?

Nurse: Well, you don't have to decide straight away. Have you asked anyone else about it?

Joan: There's no one I can talk to about this – it's all up to me I suppose.

Nurse: How do you usually decide things like this?

Joan: I don't often have to deal with things like this.

Nurse: How could you start to decide?

Joan: I suppose I could think about the bad things and the good things about taking the drugs, or not taking the drugs.

Nurse: That would be a start. So – what are the things that worry you about taking them?

This is another difficult example of what nurses have to handle – in this case the 'aftermath' of a doctor's interaction with the patient. Here Joan is trying to get the nurse to give an opinion on whether or not she should commit to a course of medication that may have significant side effects. The probability is that the nurse has got an opinion and it may even be a very strong opinion. But she keeps it to herself. You can see that despite being pressed for an opinion she keeps the decision-making with Joan. This is empowering in the sense that when Joan does eventually make a decision, it is likely that this is one she has made herself, using her own rationality and reason. What the nurse is doing is helping Joan in this process, directing her towards a decision-making process that is comfortable and familiar.

And a final example:

Nurse: Hi, Mrs Finnegan. Have you managed to persuade your daughter to let us have a look at that thing in her eye? She's not very keen is she?

Mrs Finnegan: She was in hospital last year when she fell off her bike and banged her head. It's scary when you're five.

Nurse: Yes, I know. We need to have a look soon though. If she keeps rubbing it, she may do some damage.

Mrs Finnegan: Why don't you talk to her? She doesn't seem to take any notice of me. I wish her dad was here. He's never around when I want him for things like this.

Nurse: Would he be able to help?

Mrs Finnegan: Well, he's much calmer than me, usually, and Rachael adores him.

Nurse: Is there any way we could do that?

Mrs Finnegan: I could try his mobile. Maybe he'd talk to her on the phone. I didn't think of that.

This is yet another demonstration of the nurse facilitating the person through a basic problem-solving cycle, i.e. identifying the problem and a course of action to try out until the problem is resolved or the nature of the problem changes (Egan 2002).

Reflective activity

Review the above situations. Think of similar ones that you've experienced in your practice. How were they resolved? What is empowering language? Give examples. What is disempowering language? Give examples.

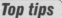

Top tips

One way to get into using a more empowering approach is to try to be more empathic with patients, relatives and colleagues that you meet in your work situations (Rogers 1967, Bonham 2004). How does it feel to be them? Can you tell them accurately that you have some idea of what they might be experiencing?

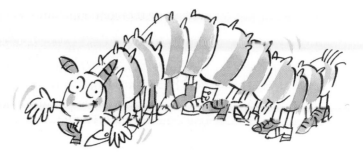

Try stepping into my shoes.

> ## Over to you
>
> Read again the section on empathy in Chapter 3 and try to demonstrate this quality in practice. Think carefully about how you do it. Make sure you discuss this with a more experienced member of staff so that you obtain helpful feedback.

Key points

- Use empowering language to encourage self determination and decision making of others
- Help the patient to help themselves

Stigmatising language

Keywords

Stigma
A label or mark that is associated with disgrace or undermines a person's character or identity

We need to take care to avoid the use of labels or descriptions that isolate, belittle or are abusive to others. Sometimes this is obvious, for example, in referring to someone as 'schizophrenic' or 'nutter', 'retarded' or 'dim', 'obese' or 'fat', but often we don't even realise how the way we talk or write about others might create **stigma** (Bowers 1998). For example, the following statement appears straightforward and neutral at first: 'He has lots of allergies. He is sensitive to everything.' But on closer examination, you can see the potential for belittlement here with the connotation that the individual is purposefully collecting or even perhaps inventing allergies, and promotes a sense that he may be over-sensitive or flawed in some way at a psychological level. The names of care environments themselves can act as stigmatising labels. Imagine overhearing someone saying 'He has been referred to. . .' and then adding one of the following: learning disabilities, psychiatry, sexual disease or memory clinic and so on. What might you think of the person just from that limited information? What might such labels mean to people who are cared for in these settings or to their significant others? This is another difficult area for nurses and other health care workers. We try to avoid stigmatising language but in some ways it helps us recognise, as professionals, the area we are trying to manage. The downside of stigmatising language is the way that it can cause us to make incorrect or inaccurate assumptions about the people we are caring for, to the detriment of their care.

Reflective activity

Consider the following three statements:

'*She is very challenging in terms of her problems. We've already identified that she abuses alcohol and non-prescription drugs. Her kids are in and out of care. She self harms regularly and turns up at A and E. Her partner is violent towards her.*'

'*He's fallen in with the wrong crowd again – despite all the work we did with him while he was on the unit. He does nothing all day but sleep, drink in his room and mess about on his computer. Then at night he goes out to meet his so-called friends and wanders the streets causing havoc with the neighbours, apparently. His mother phoned the other day to ask us why we wouldn't admit him again. She was being quite aggressive and very unreasonable – but that's her, isn't it?*'

'*She's really cranky especially towards night-time. I think it's called 'sundowning'. She gets very agitated and wanders around the ward. It's very difficult for us as we're so short-staffed here. She winds up the other patients. One of them actually hit her yesterday. And then there's the soiling . . . '*

How many stigmatising terms can you find in these descriptions? What is the mental picture or image you have of the individuals? If you met them, what would be your attitude towards them? Develop the assumptions you make based on the descriptions above. Where do these assumptions take you? Consider how the language that is used in the descriptions affects what you think about the individuals.

You can see from the statements in the reflective activity how the images that come to mind, as you hear the story, are difficult to resist. As indicated above, some of these images are useful to the professional carer. They provide a compressed way of summing up a patient quickly and succinctly. But compression of the story can bring distortion, bias, assumption, stereotyping – and ultimately, stigma. In other words, assumptions drive or lead the care that is given, rather than care being guided by **objectivity** and fact.

⊶ᴛ *Keywords*

Objectivity
A view of things that is factual, free of emotion and value judgement

> ## Reflective activity
>
> Think of occasions in practice where you have become aware of your own or others' use of stigmatising language. What other language might have been used in its place? What effect, if any, did the use of this language have on colleagues, patients, relatives?

> ## Over to you
>
> Try to spot when stigmatising communication is being used in your work place. It is probably more common than you think. Note down alternative expressions that reduce or eliminate stigma. Use a reflective diary or work book. Make sure that you maintain confidentiality by disguising any scenarios you use, even if they are intended for your own use only.

Giving feedback

Giving feedback to others should be constructive not destructive and facilitate positive change. As with many other aspects of communication discussed in this book, this is not always easy or straightforward. To be able to do this consistently takes a high level of empathy with the person who is the recipient of your feedback. The reason for this is that the best judge of what is constructive and facilitative of change is the person for whom the feedback is intended. It is unlikely, however, that they will think of your interventions in these terms.

An example of how this might work is the patient who is resistant to the care being provided. Consider Charlotte, who is a secretary. She has been off work for several months while recovering from a road accident. She needed surgery after she was knocked down by a hit and run driver. Since the surgery she has needed intensive physiotherapy treatment. She has also been referred to psychiatric services as she experiences flashbacks and nightmares about the accident. She is being seen today by the district nurse who is checking the progress of a particularly deep wound in her ankle that is only healing slowly. Note how the district nurse is attempting to give feedback that is 'constructive' and which 'facilitates positive change'. Another way of interpreting what she is doing could be described quite simply as being 'supportive' (Heron 2001).

Charlotte: It seems to be taking forever, doesn't it?

Nurse: It's slow, yes. But think what it was like only two months ago. Another few weeks and you'll see that it'll be different again.

Charlotte: Yes, I suppose I'll be left with a massive scar. I don't know what my boyfriend will think. He's so image conscious.

Nurse: I know what you're saying, but if you think back, Dave's been really supportive all along, hasn't he? And it's difficult to say what your ankle will look like until the tissue has repaired a little more. It takes time, doesn't it?

You'll be aware that sometimes encouraging interventions that are intended to support and reassure work i.e. the patient feels supported and reassured. However, at other times they don't work and the patient will not be reassured, although they may feel supported. That said, it is part of our professional role to be *realistically* optimistic (Bonham 2004) and positive, when we discuss the future with the patient:

Charlotte: Yes, I know it takes time, but I'm still going to look awful, aren't I?

Nurse: It's impossible to say. I've seen quite a few wounds fairly similar to this. In my experience I think you'll be surprised at how good the body is at recovery and disguise. It's important that you exercise gently as the physiotherapist suggested. There are other things as well such as maintaining your healthy diet and keeping off cigarettes, just like you were doing before the accident.

Here is another example:

Nurse: Edith, how are you this morning? It's a lovely day out there. Look at the colours on those trees. Did you have a good sleep last night?

Edith: Who are you? Go away! Where's my husband? Somebody slept in my bed again last night. I'm calling the police.

Nurse: Edith, I was here all night looking after you. You slept in your own bed all night. Bill will be here this afternoon. He always comes to see you on Sundays, doesn't he? Look at those trees, aren't they beautiful?

Edith: What time is Bill coming? What's the time now? Where's my hairbrush? I want to do my hair.

Nurse: Good idea, Edith!

You will be aware that the patient here seems to be confused. The reason is not clear, and doesn't matter in terms of this example. Throughout, the nurse remains rooted in the real world without being confrontational. She diverts Edith into positive activity and the real things that are happening in Edith's world. She is, again, positive, optimistic, constructive and supportive. She tries to avoid reinforcing Edith's confusion.

And a third example:

Nurse: How did you get on with that admission, Naomi?

Naomi (a student nurse): Well, not too bad I suppose. I couldn't really get much from her. She doesn't seem to want to talk much. I had to keep finding where I was on the admission forms as well, which didn't help.

Nurse: How does she seem though?

Naomi: Well, when I was showing her around she gave me a bit of eye contact and smiled once. She kept asking when she could have a cigarette. She seems to know some of the other patients here. She asked if I was on duty again tomorrow. I don't really know what to make of her.

Nurse: So what are you going to do next?

Naomi: Well, I've given her a drink in the day room. I said I'd see her again in an hour just to try to do a bit more. She seemed OK about that. I'll just keep an eye on her until then. Oh, I've asked Annie to sit with her for a while as well as she remembers her from the last admission. I thought that might help.

Nurse: So – you're well on the way with the admission paperwork. You've given the patient a drink and shown her around. She's recognised some people she knows and you've put someone with her to make sure she's OK. You'll continue with her later on today, and she knows that. Sounds good to me, Naomi. You'll get used to the paperwork with repetition. The main thing now is that the patient is safe, observed and reasonably comfortable. You seem to have done all that. Well done!

The nurse has **validated** and supported the actions of the student nurse who actually doesn't realise that she's been effective in terms of the outcomes she's achieved during the admission.

Keywords

Validate
Confirm, support, encourage

Reflective activity

How many times do *you* receive this kind of feedback? How do you feel when you get it? How do you feel when you don't? How important is it that patients receive it? Think of occasions when you have given patients or colleagues constructive and facilitating feedback. Think of occasions when you might have missed the opportunity.

Key points **Top tips**

An effective way to get a little nearer to providing constructive and positive feedback to an individual is to take a little time to consider the person 'in the round', gaining a sense of what the world might be like from their point of view, then demonstrating empathy.

Over to you

Try to integrate this style of nursing into your everyday practice. It's not just for special occasions. The more you try this form of communicating, the more it will become part of you, and in turn, the less you will need to think about it.

Key points Top tips

Constructive feedback:

● requires a high level of empathy
● facilitates positive change
● validates the contribution of others

Receiving feedback

Just as it is important to consider giving feedback, we should also consider how to receive and give appropriate consideration to feedback from service users, carers, relatives and colleagues. In the ideal world we would, as professional carers, respond positively to feedback from any recipients of our care and anyone else who is connected with that care. After all, we want the best for our patients don't we? Consider the feedback we may get from patients and how we might respond to it:

Dave: Nurse, any chance of a chat later? I've been feeling a bit down since my parents went. You know how they wind me up – especially mum.

Nurse: I'm sorry, Dave. We're expecting a new admission shortly. I won't be able to talk with you tonight. I'm off for a couple of days then. You could always talk to one of the other staff. They all know you pretty well.

Dave: I wanted to talk to you. You're the only one I can really open up to. You really seem to understand me. I can't talk to my girlfriend like I can talk to you. You're the best nurse on this ward.

Nurse: Thanks, it's nice of you to say that, but I really can't do it tonight.

Dave: Oh, please yourself then. I won't bother asking again.

This feedback seems very complimentary, at first. The patient has singled out the nurse as having the greatest understanding of his problems. In fact, she's better than any of her colleagues! When she reasonably redirects him to a colleague, because she has a more pressing business to deal with, he seems to react badly. What could be the reasons for this? How could the nurse have managed this reaction? What else might be happening in terms of Dave's relationship with the nurse?

Consider this scenario next:

Nurse: Hello, can I help you?

Mr Clements: I'd like to speak to the nurse in charge.

Nurse: Yes, that's me.

Mr Clements: Have you seen the state of my mother? This is the third time I've visited her and she hasn't got her teeth in, she's got food spilt down her dress, and the dress isn't even hers. What the hell is going on?

Nurse: Right, I don't know how that's happened. Have a seat in the office, just here, Mr Clements. I'll go and talk to the nurse who's in charge of your mother's care. Give me a minute or two?

Mr Clements: I need to go soon. I've ordered a taxi. I'll be writing to the hospital managers about this. I'm sick of this place.

What else can the nurse do to manage this difficult situation? What should she do when Mr Clements has left? Consider what circumstances may have led up to Mr Clements' complaint.

Here is a third example:

Doctor Miller: Nurse, have those blood results come back yet for Mrs Niles?

Nurse: I'm not sure. I'll go and check. They hadn't arrived at handover.

Doctor Miller: Those bloody lab people want a good shaking. How long does it take? We never had this problem at Guy's.

Nurse: Found them. They'd been put in her notes.

Doctor Miller: Who the hell did that? Is this ward staffed by idiots? I've been asking for these results since yesterday morning. Was it that student? He seems to be on another planet!

The positive part of this scenario is that Mrs Niles' blood test results have been received and found. Probably the student thought that he was doing the right thing by putting them in her notes. Is the doctor reacting in a reasonable manner? What might be the circumstances that underlie his behaviour? How might the nurse react to his outburst in a positive and constructive way?

And here is a fourth example:

Mr Clements: Hello, Sister. Can a have a word?

Ward Sister: Sure, Mr. Clements. Do you want to come down to the office for a minute?

Mr Clements: I just wanted to apologise for my behaviour the other day – with your colleague. I'm sure she must have told you about it?

Sister: Yes, she passed it on to me. We checked what had happened that shift with your mother. I understand that the hospital manager has written to you about it.

Mr Clements: I got the letter yesterday. Most of what I said was uncalled for, although I was angry about the state of her teeth. Really, I'm very grateful for what you've done for my mother on this ward. I'd like to show my appreciation to your staff. I was wondering if I could make a donation to the ward. Perhaps you could use it to take everyone out for a meal? My brother owns the Highroads Restaurant in town. We could arrange something? What do you think?

As with the first example, in the above section, this appears to be complimentary. How should the Ward Sister respond to Mr Clements' generosity? Can you foresee any problems with the offer, or is it as straightforward as it seems? Can you give any explanation for Mr Clements' apparent about-turn in his attitude to the ward staff?

Reflective activity

What examples from your practice experience can you recall that are similar to the examples above? How were they handled by the nursing staff (or others if appropriate)? What was the history to the situations that you recall? Are there any themes that might link the scenarios above and your experiences in real life practice? What are some of the things that cause people to give feedback to us as nurses? What about the people who never give us any feedback at all? Do we assume that they are happy and satisfied with the service we are providing?

If we don't get feedback from our clients and their relatives and other professionals, should we ask for it? If so, how do we do that? What would we do with the results? What feedback mechanisms, if any, have you seen in your practice? Are they used effectively? What is the impact of their use on patient care? What have you learnt from these situations?

Key points **Top tips**

Never dismiss *any* feedback about the service that you and your colleagues provide. All feedback is useful, but some kinds may be more difficult to make sense of than others. Discuss with your colleagues what, if any, action needs to be taken after feedback has been received.

Over to you

Do you have any structured methods of analysing feedback or recording it? What about compliments and thanks from patients and relatives? What about complaints? What about comments that are seen as complaints but might be intended to be helpful by the sender?

Key points Top tips

- Feedback should be welcomed from service users, carers, relatives, and colleagues

Giving information, teaching and promoting health

The role of the nurse is diverse and, alongside providing clinical care, extends to being a teacher, health promoter and giver of information. This much broader level of activity and involvement is described by Mackintosh (1996) as involving 'social, economic and political change to ensure that the environment is conducive to health. Health promotion not only encompasses a nurse educating an individual about his health needs, but also demands that the nurse plays her part in attempting to address the wider environmental and social issues that adversely affect people's health' (p. 14). Whitehead (2003) provides some useful guidance in terms of effective health communication in educating others (Box 4.1).

Record keeping

These days being a nurse involves using a variety of documents, such as procedure manuals, nursing policies, and the nursing process itself. Like doctors, nurses keep their own records to formally establish or constitute the reality of care in their own terms and direct subsequent nursing action to deal with that reality. These

Box 4.1: Health education tips

- Determine individual learning styles, adopting a flexible approach to presentation of material to suit the individual learner, small or large group, using exercises and activities where possible to increase learner involvement and aid memory for what was taught
- Establish and maintain effective learning environments, paying attention to noise levels, but also being flexible and creative in teaching 'on the hoof' alongside busy clinical activities
- It is best to set out learning objectives and outcomes for any teaching, paying attention to time limits and resources, delivering content in small chunks with sufficient breaks
- Use appropriate resources to support learning such as PowerPoint, audio-visual materials, the Internet, and so on
- Provide handouts for any session, with suggested reading, and follow-up questions
- Evaluate the teaching session, especially whether it is leading to changes in the clients' health status

(Adapted from Whitehead 2003)

records underpin the working relationship between nurses and patients. One way of gaining insight into the importance of such records is to imagine what would happen if all such documents in all hospitals and health centres were to vanish overnight!

Berg (1996) demonstrates that health care records achieve a 'semi-public memory' of the work that is done and helps to organise and 'keep track' of this activity. This is true of medical and nursing records. If you like, each record is a 'structured distributing and collecting device', where all tasks concerning a patient's care begins and ends. As Berg (1996) puts it: 'The simple ticking of a box, or the jotting down of some words set organisational routines in motion' (p. 510). The records, therefore, enable staff to make sense of their patients.

Reflective activity

Record keeping is often repetitive and not always patient centred. It is worth thinking about health care records at different levels: organisational policy requirements; design of forms or computer data entry systems; kinds of descriptions of patients which are entered; the way the records are used; how patients can be encouraged to say the right things to the health care professionals so as to influence what they write; the current use of patient centred multidisciplinary records; audited care pathways.

- Review the type of record keeping you have observed
- Make a few critical comments about how records are compiled or used

◉━┰ *Keywords*

Repositories
Places where things are stored

Berg (1996) highlights the 'paper life' of health care organisations – the way that it is dependent on documentation. In this sense records are seen as public **repositories**, which store the actions of professionals for inspection or auditing.

Generally speaking, once all the interactions with patients or clients have been undertaken, the next stage for many health care professionals is to make some account of what took place. Increasingly, with the implementation of the Electronic Patient Records (EPR) and Electronic Health Records (EHR) (Department of Health 2000) such information is being created, stored and disseminated electronically. In addition to providing information for day-to-day clinical care, records serve a role in resource management, self evaluation, audits of performance, care, quality assurance and research (Currell and Wainwright 1996). Yet the Audit Commission (1999) has criticised the poor standard of NHS record keeping and recommended that action should be taken to remedy this. But despite the report and the call for high quality records in the nursing literature (Pennels 2002), and Allen's (1998) finding that nursing staff were positive about record keeping in general because of its link with the nursing process and because it represented professionalism, there is good evidence that health professionals are not adhering to guidelines and failing to include such elementary information as the date or whether important diagnostic information has been taken into account (Sharma *et al*, 2002.)

Howse and Bailey (1992) found that nurses do not always have confidence in their writing skills and struggle to put into words what exactly is done in nursing practice. This difficulty is part of a wider difficulty in capturing in words the complex reality of any event or activity, whether it is in health care or not. Adding more and more detail does not necessarily improve matters. In fact, excessive detail may suggest that the writer or speaker is trying to be convincing. It does not necessarily correspond to what you would have seen if you had been there in the first place. Therefore, the drive towards accuracy and completeness can only take us so far. Indeed, Moloney and Maggs (1999) found that despite high levels of investment in record keeping and care planning, there was little evidence that such systems led to better patient outcomes. This supports an earlier report by Marr *et al.* (1993) who found that bedside terminals may be scarcely used and a later study by Sharma *et al.* (2002) who identify major omissions in detail.

Perhaps one way to improve the situation, as highlighted by Crow and Harmeling (2002), involves redesigning records to reflect the assessment procedures that practitioners use, and correspond to the way they deal with their patients. Thus the information is collected in a way which is intuitive and fits easily into the diagnostic and treatment process, rather than seeming like an extra burden.

Increasingly, as part of the modernisation agenda in the NHS in the UK, patients are considered partners in care and it is now a common view that recording care should be, where possible, a joint venture. This is surely a positive step in achieving a meaningful record of care.

Also, the recording and communication of care is a rapidly changing field. Currently, there is a national NHS programme for better information for health called 'Connecting for Health' that will assist in documentation through electronic health records and care pathways. This will bring modern computer systems into the NHS, which will improve patient care and services over the next ten years. As their website notes: 'The NHS is changing the way it works. Its vision for the future is to have a more modern, efficient, patient-led health service and to give patients more choice and control over their own health and care.' At the heart of this initiative is the NHS Care Records Service which is aiming to improve the sharing of patients' records across the NHS with their consent, making communication much easier between GPs and hospital services, including the provision of electronic prescriptions.

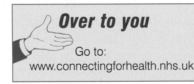

Over to you

Go to:
www.connectingforhealth.nhs.uk

Professional accountability and record keeping

Although there are problems with record keeping, not least with patterns of care being so complex that the record is only ever a partial account of what has occurred in order to ensure the legal adequacy of records in the UK, the Nursing and Midwifery Council (NMC) (2002) recommends that they include the following:

- *a full account of your assessment and the care you have planned and provided*
- *relevant information about the condition of the patient or client at any given time and the measures you have taken to respond to their needs*
- *evidence that you have understood and honoured your duty of care, that you have taken all reasonable steps to care for the*

patient or client and that any actions or omissions on your part have not compromised their safety in any way

● *a record of any arrangements you have made for the continuing care of a patient or client.*

The NMC does not stipulate the frequency of entries as these will be determined by professional judgement, local standards and agreements. It recommends more careful and detailed reporting when 'patients or clients present complex problems, show deviation from the norm, require more intensive care than normal, are confused and disoriented or generally give cause for concern. You must use your professional judgement (if necessary in discussion with other members of the health care team) to determine when these circumstances exist' (Nursing and Midwifery Council 2002, p. 9).

Reflective activity

Examine nursing entries in patient records:

● Can you find examples of 'weak' entries that provide little information such as 'No problems', 'Appears fine', 'No change'?

● Why are 'weak' entries made? What factors influence the way nurses make entries in records?

● What kinds of records would be more useful?

Over to you

Go to:
www.nmc-uk.org

In a similar way to the NMC's guidelines, the International Council of Nurses (1999) offers three key elements to describing activities in nursing. They suggest that records should include:

1. Nursing phenomena or nursing diagnoses
2. Nursing actions or nursing interventions, and
3. Nursing outcomes (Kisilowska 2001).

While nurses, like everyone else, can never guarantee the meanings of their written words, they need to remain vigilant in reducing the scope for misinterpretation of people in their care. The

Key points **Top tips**

When authorised to record care:

● Stick to the facts, such as evidence from observations etc.
● Avoid rambling, overlong description
● Do not make general comments that judge an individual's character or personality
● Do not use language that is likely to offend
● Where possible, report significant statements from patients word-for-word using quotation marks
● Where possible and appropriate check key information with the patient or client and supervisor
● Avoid vague comments such as 'making progress', 'had a good day', 'appears well', etc.
● Attend to legal, formal requirements for completing paper or electronic records

⚬━┭ Keywords

Incarcerate
Imprision or confine

Incapacitate
To render a person unfit or incapable

power of language to construct the world in which we live makes it important for nurses to monitor health care language as it affects the lives of others. Effective nursing practice involves a critical interest in how we write about those in our care, how other professionals write about them, or how patients are enabled to account for themselves in records. Effectively, caring involves vigilant communication in patient records.

In writing, we should be concerned about how health care professionals represent those in their care and whether they **incarcerate**, **incapacitate** or restrain them in reality by using judgemental words and phrases and even reaching conclusions that may be false and damage the reputation or standing of the patient or client. In other words, records can confine, limit or negatively affect the lives of patients. For example, a GP's referral letter to a Community Mental Health Nurse described a client as a 'young prostitute' with an 'inadequate personality'. On visiting the client at home, there was no evidence that she was either a 'prostitute' or 'inadequate', but had merely complained of tiredness (Crawford *et al*. 1995). If this report had gone unchallenged, the individual may have been severley disadvantaged. This incident highlights the need to oppose communication that we consider prejudicial, damaging or unethical. But more than this, it reminds us not to believe everything that is written down or reported to us!

So, in summary, we have learned that completing records is not always straightforward and that there are a number of limitations to the whole process – not least in misrepresenting real flesh and blood individuals. The official guidelines only go so far in showing nurses how to complete written reports. What is required is for nurses to develop a keen sense of how what is written about another person can have negative consequences, for example, influencing decision-making about the status of an individual on a section of the Mental Health Act (1983). This ethical vigilance should be at the heart of reflective practice and our role as advocates – that is, working on behalf of the patients or clients (Grace 2001), or if you prefer, being 'one who pleads, intercedes or speaks for or on behalf of, another' (*The Oxford English Dictionary* 1989, p. 194).

> ### Over to you
>
> Read:
> Teasdale, K. (1998) *Advocacy in Health Care*. Blackwell Science, Oxford.

Confidentiality and access to records

In the UK, a good many records are kept about patients in a wide variety of locations. For example, an individual's records might be lodged at a GP's surgery, held by health visitors or district nurses, at the hospitals they attend, and so on, emerging in different forms through their lifetime (Williams *et al.* 1993). As the Audit Commission (1999) found, these records are often difficult to use because they were: incomplete; and structured in a variety of different ways with only half of them having any kind of index or guide to the contents. This makes the information difficult to navigate for the user. Indeed, some clinicians appeared to spend as much as 20 per cent of their time at work locating information in records.

Beyond the issue of the variable and unsatisfactory nature of records, the question arises about what kind of information from such records should be disclosed to different professional groups. The Caldicott Report (Department of Health 1997) raised a number of concerns about the general lack of awareness of confidentiality and information security requirements throughout the NHS at all levels. It was also concerned that the NHS could limit access to patient information to those who truly need to know.

Everyone working for or with the NHS who records, handles, stores or otherwise comes across patient information has a personal common law duty of confidence to patients and to his or her employer (Department of Health 2002). This duty of confidence continues even after the death of the patient or after an employee or contractor has left the NHS. The duty of confidence to an employer regarding company/NHS Trust information is included in the terms and conditions of employment and breaches of confidentiality in relation to individual patients and/or of NHS Trust information can result in disciplinary procedures being taken against the employee (Data Protection Act 1998). The patient too can take legal action against the individual within the remit of negligence in a 'Duty of Care' (McHale *et al.* 1998).

If you are considering conducting research using patients records, approval must first be sought from a Local Research Ethics Committee (LREC). Three areas have special regulations: information relating to sexually transmitted diseases (including HIV and AIDS); human fertilisation; and abortions.

Access to records by patients

Following the Access to Health Records Act (1990), Data Protection Act (1998) and Human Rights Act (2000) patients are permitted access to all manual health records whenever made, subject to specified exceptions. This freeing of information has been further enhanced by a culture of partnership whereby the patient is included in all correspondence between a hospital consultant and the patient's GP (the 'copy letters' project) and allowing patients to browse their own records on a computer terminal (NHS 2003).

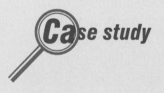

Case study

You read the following entry by a colleague in a patient's nursing record:
'*John is a manipulative individual who will do anything to get attention. He thinks he is God's gift to women and struts about like a peacock. He is rude and has a big personal hygiene problem.*'

As you are reading the entry, John enters the office, sees that you are looking at his notes and asks what you find so interesting. He requests to look at the document, stating: 'I'd like to know what you lot are writing about me.'

● What is your immediate response?
● What further actions would you recommend?

Key points   Top tips

Care records:
● underpin the working relationship between nurses and patients
● enable staff to make sense of their patients
● are increasingly created, stored and disseminated electronically
● may disadvantage or misrepresent patients
● are subject to professional and legal requirements and standards concerning security, confidentiality and access.

RRRRRRapid recap

Check your progress so far by working though each of the following questions:

1. What word refers to reaching a harmonious agreement?
2. What is another word for a label or mark that is associated with disgrace or undermines a person's character or identity?
3. Berg (1996) refers to health care records as a 'semi-public' what?
4. Which professional body requires that nurses provide 'relevant information about the condition of the patient or client at any given time and the measures you have taken to respond to their needs'?
5. Which three Acts of Parliament permit access by patients to all manual health records whenever made, subject to specified exceptions?

If you have difficulty with more than one of the questions, read through the section again to refresh your understanding before moving on.

References

Allen, D. (1998) Record keeping and routine nursing practice: The view from the wards. *Journal of Advanced Nursing*, **27**, 1223–1230.

Audit Commission (1999) *Setting the Record Straight. A review of progress in health records services.* Audit Commission Publications, London.

Berg, M. (1996) Practices of reading and writing: The constitutive role of the patient record in medical work. *Sociology of Health and Illness*, **18**(4) 499–524.

Bonham, P. (2004) *Communicating as a Mental Health Carer.* Nelson Thornes, Cheltenham.

Bowers, L. (1998) *The Social Nature of Mental Illness.* Routledge, London.

Crawford, P., Nolan, P. and Brown, B. (1995) Linguistic entrapment: Medico-nursing biographies as fictions. *Journal of Advanced Nursing*, **22**, 1141–1148.

Crow, J.L. and Harmeling, B.C. (2002) Development of a consensus and evidence based standardised clinical assessment ands record form for neurological inpatients. *Physiotherapy*, **88**(1), 33–46.

Currell, R. and Wainwright, P. (1996) Nursing record systems, nursing practice and patient care (Protocol). In: *Collaboration on Effective Professional Practice Module of the Cochrane Database of Systematic Reviews* (eds Bero, L., Grilli, R., Grimshaw, J. and Oxman, A.). The Cochrane Collaboration, Oxford, pp. 47–61.

De Bono, E. (1973) *Lateral Thinking: Creativity Step by Step.* Harper Paperbacks, London.

Department of Health (1997) *The Caldicott Committee: a report on the review of patient-identifiable information.* Department of Health, London.

Department of Health (2000) *Good practice guidelines for general practice electronic patient records.* www.doh.gov.uk/gpepr/guidelines.pdf (accessed 24/5/2003).

Department of Health (2002) *Statutory instrument 2002 no. 1438 The Health Service (control of patient information) regulations* www.doh.gov.uk/ipu/confiden/instrument.pdf (accessed 24/5/2003)

Egan, G. (2002) *The Skilled Helper*, 7th edn. Brooks Cole, Pacific Grove, CA.

Grace, P.J. (2001) Professional advocacy: Widening the scope of accountability. *Nursing Philosophy*, **2**, 151–162.

Heron, J. (2001) *Helping the Client*, 5th edn. Sage, London.

Howse, E. and Bailey, J. (1992) Resistance to documentation: A nursing research issue. *International Journal of Nursing Studies*, **29**(4), 371–381.

International Council of Nurses (1999) *International Classification for Nursing practice (beta version)*. International Council of Nurses, Geneva.

Kisilowska, M. (2001) Reorganized structure and other proposals for the ICNP development. *International Nursing Review* **4**, 218–233.

Mackintosh, N. (1996) *Promoting health: An issue for nursing*. Quay Books, Dinton.

Marr, P.B., Duthie, E., Glassman, K.S., Janovas, D.M., Kelly, J.B., Graham, E., Kovner, C.T., Rienzei, A., Roberts, N.K. and Schick, D. (1993) Bedside terminals and quality of nursing documentation. *Computers in Nursing*, **11**(4), 176–182.

McHale, J., Tingle, J. and Peysner, J. (1998) *Law and Nursing.* Butterworth Heinemann, Oxford.

Moloney, R. and Maggs, C. (1999) A systematic review of the relationships between written manual nursing care planning, record keeping and patient outcomes. *Journal of Advanced Nursing*, **30**(1), 51–57.

NHS (2003) *IT questions and answers* www.nhs.uk/nhsmagazine/primarycare/it_qa.asp (accessed 24/5/2003).

Nursing and Midwifery Council (2002) *Code of Conduct*. Nursing and Midwifery Council, London.

Nursing and Midwifery Council (2002) *Guidelines for Records and Record Keeping*. Nursing and Midwifery Council, London.

Pennels, C. (2002) The importance of accurate and comprehensive record keeping. *Professional Nurse*, **17**(5), 294–296.

Sharma, S., Downey, G. and Heywood, R. (2002) Guidelines: Are they adhered to in clinical practice? *Journal of Clinical Governance*, **10**(2), 71–75.

Teasdale, K. (1998) *Advocacy in Health Care*. Blackwell Science, Oxford.

Watkins, P. (2001) *Mental Health Nursing: The art of compassionate care*. Butterworth Heinemann, Oxford.

Whitehead, D. (2003) Evaluating health promotion: A model for nursing practice, *Journal of Advanced Nursing*, **41**(5), 490–498.

Williams, J.G., Roberts, R. and Rigby, M.J. (1993) Integrated patient records: Another move towards quality for patients. *Quality in Health Care*, **2**(2), 73–74.

Rogers, C. R. (1967) *On Becoming a Person*. Constable & Robinson, London.

Managing challenging communication

Learning outcomes

By the end of this chapter you should be able to:

- Identify, explain and clarify the causes of conflict or challenge that occur in health care
- Describe skills and best practice for communicating in challenging situations or during conflict or complaint that may result in violence or aggression, especially the use of verbal and non-verbal de-escalation
- Describe best practice in dealing with complaints and reducing hostility in telephone enquiries such as identifying oneself, being polite, striving to reduce hostility or conflict, resolving queries or concerns
- Describe best practice in breaking bad news
- Consider the impact or effect of anxiety, stress or depression on communication and identify strategies to enhance interaction
- Consider the communication needs of people who do not speak English or where English is their second language

Introduction

This chapter discusses a range of challenges to communication and offers practical guidance for resolution that is based on current evidence about dealing with challenging behaviour or aggression; with complaints; and breaking bad news.

We will discuss management of challenging situations that may result in conflict. This includes an examination of the triggers for conflict and handling potential conflict effectively by attention to attitudes, behaviours, verbal and non-verbal communication strategies. Theoretical frameworks that help us understand what is happening in conflict situations will be discussed.

The causes of conflict and challenge in health care settings are infinite. In this section only a few will be identified and discussed, together with some related communication strategies that might help. For more breadth in this area the reader is advised to look at additional texts such as Harrison and Hart (2006), Mason and Chandley (1999), Marelli (1997) and Gillies (1994).

Dealing with the disgruntled patient

A common cause of patients becoming frustrated then irritated, and perhaps even angry, is the way that the professional carers around them apparently fail to communicate effectively. Or sometimes it can be the style and content of the carer's communication that starts to cause problems. This sometimes escalates into unnecessary difficulties. The carer can be completely oblivious of the effect that they may be having on the patient, as can be seen from this example:

Nurse: Mr Bowles, you can stop buzzing now. We heard it ten minutes ago. Can I help?

Mr Bowles: It's too late. I've just thrown up again. I couldn't get to the toilet. I knew it was going to happen.

Nurse: Never mind. I'll be back in a minute. I'll clear you up then.

Mr. Bowles: I'm fed up with you lot on this ward. You're always saying I'll be back in a minute. I bet I won't see you until tomorrow morning. The night staff will be sorting me out again.

It is probably clear to you, from your practice experience, that this kind of interchange between nurse and patient almost always has a history to it. The patient is building up a set of experiences that tell him that the staff on the ward don't do what they say they will do. The nurse is using a clichéd approach that has appeared to work in the past. 'I'll be back in a minute' is being used as a delaying tactic to give the nurse some space to reassess, plan and cope with a constantly fluctuating work load.

Sometimes, however, the patient can bring their problems into a health care environment with them and you can become an unwitting scapegoat for the expression of their feelings about this. For example:

Nurse: Good evening, Mrs Kane. Did your husband come to see you again, this afternoon?

Mrs Kane: No, he bloody didn't! If he calls, tell him to get lost!

Here you see the nurse being on the receiving end of a different form of a patient's exasperation. The question is how can this exasperation be addressed by *thoughtful* use of communication on the part of nurse? In both examples we are dealing with 'flashpoints' – a build up of frustration on the part of the patient. Some ways of perhaps avoiding this (not guaranteed!) are as follows:

1. Be aware of the affect of patients. What is their usual mood like? Is it different today? How is it different? Why is it different?

You may already know this from other staff:

'Dennis is much brighter today. The doctor told him he could go home at the weekend.'

'Alan is a bit flat this morning. The admission last night was really noisy and he couldn't get back to sleep.'

'I've noticed Jane's very agitated this afternoon. I think her mum is visiting tonight. She always gets like this.'

If, however, you are not picking up this information from colleagues, a useful response is to check it for yourself. This, of course, can be very simple and direct, or it can take a considerable level of skill.

Nurse: Hi, Dennis. You're looking brighter this morning. What's happened?

Dennis: Great news! I can try a weekend at home. I can't wait!

Keywords

Affect
The mood or emotional presentation of a person, e.g. 'flat in affect' means flattened mood

Nurse: Alan, how are you doing? You look really down.
Alan: Oh, it's OK thanks. I'm just exhausted. All that racket last night. I'm shattered.

Nurse: Come and sit down, Jane. Let's have a cuppa. What's happening now?
Jane: My bloody mother! She's doing it to me again.

Notice how the use of an open questioning technique can often be very helpful (Bonham 2004).

2. Be aware of the patient's non-verbal communication. How do they usually look? Do they look different today? How do they look different? What made you notice the difference in the first place?

As above, this information may come from others, or you may be the first one to notice:

'Madge looks like she's just got out of bed and it's nearly lunch time. She's usually really smart. Do you think she's OK?'

'Have you noticed Bill? I don't think that jacket belongs to him. Look, it's far too short. I found him in someone else's room yesterday. I wonder what's happening?'

'Jenny! You look great. You've got some lipstick on! It makes you look really different!'

Of course this is just the first stage. The second stage is turning this new information into useful nursing data which can be used to help the patient. Again, the use of *gentle, tentative* questioning can sometimes help to reveal new information.

Nurse: Hi, Madge. Can I get you a hairbrush and some tights? Lunch will be ready soon.
Madge: I want to see the manager now. Get me my bill, please. This hotel is a disgrace!

Nurse: Tom, I don't remember seeing you in that jacket before. Where's it from?
Tom: My son brought it in this morning. It doesn't fit me does it? I need it to keep warm though. It's freezing out there!

Nurse: So what's happening?
Jenny: My tests are all clear. I can't believe it!

3. Be aware of what the patient is saying and not saying.
Listen to what this patient is saying and not saying:

Nurse: So your son brought the jacket in for you? Didn't he notice it wasn't yours?
Tom: He didn't notice. I'm not sure he'd notice anything at the moment.

This is an important snippet of dialogue that illustrates the difference between an effective and less effective nurse. The less effective nurse is likely to ignore the patient's statement along the lines of 'Oh, right, I see.'

But the effective nurse has just been presented with what might be a very important piece of information. What is Tom saying about his son and their relationship? Is it said in jest, in seriousness, sadly, angrily? How might the nurse find out? Here are some suggestions:

'What do you mean, Tom? Do you mean he wouldn't notice anything at the moment?'

'What are you saying, Tom?'

'What do you mean?'

'I don't understand, Tom.'

The response from Tom, now that the nurse has created the opportunity, may reveal more useful information that can be used to help him.

Key points **Top tips**

Try to become more aware of the *usual* affect and non-verbal communication of patients. *Really listen* to them and check out even small changes to these usual clues by respectful, careful and tentative open style questioning. You may be surprised what you find out.

Key points Top tips

- Poor communication can lead to patients becoming frustrated, irritated and perhaps even angry
- Ways of avoiding 'flashpoints' include being aware of the affect, verbal and non-verbal communication of patients

Dealing with the dissatisfied or angry relative of a patient

It is often the lack of, or inappropriate, communication that finally triggers off dissatisfaction in the patient's relative. Sometimes, conflict can result due to issues around confidentiality. It can be very difficult, for example, to appease a frustrated visitor or telephone enquirer who wants to know what is happening to their relative but the nurse is unable to tell them anything very meaningful because of professional and organisational constraints on sharing information about patients. Most people will accept, either face to face, over the phone, or in writing, the fact that often we are unable, as nurses, to tell them very much, or maybe not everything they wish to know. The only exception to this is when the patient specifically gives permission for certain people to know certain things about them. You will probably be aware from your practice that sometimes the care team (which can be large) may know things about a patient that even very close family members do not know. It could be this very situation that causes family and friends of the patient to become so frustrated; after all, the experience of 'being kept in the dark' can be very disempowering.

Nurses can sometimes pre-empt the kind of frustrations that can arise in this situation by ensuring that the lines of communication between the patient and relatives/friends via the nursing and medical staff are made clear from the start. This would mean introducing and addressing with the patient as soon as possible after admission who they would like information shared with concerning their situation or state of health. Any decision then needs to be entered in the patient's notes to guide the communication of everyone concerned with their care. It is vital to be consistent in this matter. There are few things more likely to fuel frustration on the part of relatives and friends than being told different things by different staff. It only takes one person to be out of step for the system to look more flawed than it really is.

Reflective activity

Consider occasions when people have become angry or frustrated in your own clinical area.
   What were the triggers for this?

Key points

- The need for confidentiality can result in potential conflict with relatives making enquiries about a patient
- Nurses should ensure that the lines of communication between the patient and relatives or friends via the nursing and medical staff are made clear from the start
- There are few things more likely to fuel frustration on the part of relatives and friends than being told different things by different staff

De-escalation techniques

Of course, beyond the issue of confidentiality and information sharing, there is a great variety of situations or circumstances in clinical settings with the potential for generating frustration and anger. Health care environments can easily provoke conflict. There are lots of opportunities for interpersonal 'heat' and anger to develop. Often, a common cause for dissatisfaction is the complainant's frustration at a 'faceless' system or the breakdown of a system. For example, a distressed patient may be kept waiting for treatment and no-one from the care team is telling them how much longer they will have to wait. Or a person becomes very aggressive because no-one seems to be looking after the needs of their relative who is in great pain.

If things do go wrong, then the following steps may at least help to partially diffuse the situation:

1. Try to find a quiet space to talk with the person. The exception to this is if the person is particularly angry and possibly presenting a threat – in which case you keep within view of colleagues (see below). It is still possible to establish a feeling of privacy even in an open space where you can get help if required

2. Listen carefully to what the person is saying without interrupting.

3. Clarify and paraphrase tentatively. This will demonstrate to the person that you have understood or are trying to understand what it is that they are attempting to say

4. Avoid appearing defensive as this is likely to increase the intensity of aggression or frustration that is displayed

5. Don't take things personally and try to depersonalise issues that have resulted in conflict. A key point to remember in situations like this is that it is very unlikely (although not impossible) that the dissatisfaction being expressed is about *you* as an individual. It is most likely that you, at that particular time, are the representative of a systemic failure or an institutional failure

6. Use the person-centred techniques of trying to be empathic, accepting and congruent

7. Use a problem-solving attitude (Egan 2002), if this is feasible. Identify and clarity the problem. If there are a number of problems then try to set priorities for addressing these. Which problems can you help with realistically? Which ones can you not help with? What are the possible options or actions? Be aware that some problems that you are confronted with will be out of your area of influence, or may not be resolvable anyway

8. Make clear arrangements for the person to be referred to someone who can help them, if you know who this is, and provide information about the procedure for making complaints. Avoid appearing as if you are fobbing them off. If they suspect that you are doing this, it may cause the situation to worsen again.

As with most of the other scenarios and situations discussed in this book, the preferable tactic is to anticipate these difficult situations and try to 'nip them in the bud'. As a nurse you will often be able to 'tune in' to oncoming difficult situations and maybe discuss them with colleagues as a means of presenting a united and consistent front to the (only sometimes) unhappy people who visit our clinical areas. Or you may be able to pick up clues from the patient:

'Mum will go crazy when she finds out what's happened to our John.'

'You won't tell my husband, will you? He'll be devastated.'

'I'd prefer it if you'd tell my children that I'm going to be fine, please'.

The appropriate intervention here would be to obtain clarification of these statements made by patients, not necessarily as a separate task, but as part of the admission, part of the assessment, or part of the relationship-building process. Never be afraid to say to a patient or relative that you do not have the solution to their problem. If you are in doubt, then consult a more experienced colleague about the presented dilemma, even if this means that you have to negotiate a delay to the resolution.

Sometimes the nature of conflict in a clinical setting can be such that more immediate actions are required to protect the safety of yourself and others. If you feel under threat from the escalation of a situation with another person, the immediate consideration is your own safety. You may think that perhaps it should be the safety of the patient. Consider, however, the consequences of the patient hurting you or disabling you first, then going on to hurt themselves or others. If you protect yourself first, then you are able to get assistance to help manage the situation to reduce the chances of further injury or damage happening. This means taking the following precautions:

- Ensuring that you are not alone with a threatening person as indicated above
- If you are taken by surprise by someone who unexpectedly becomes a threat to you and you are on your own, try to make sure that you have or can create an escape route. This can be as

simple as making sure that you take up a position between the threatening person and the door

- Make sure you tell colleagues where you are going and how long you will be there, and importantly make sure they've heard you. As a routine take a personal alarm and, or, a mobile phone

- Stay in line of sight of colleagues whenever possible

- Keep back so that you are not within immediate hitting distance

- Be aware of the potential for objects to be thrown at you

- Be very aware of the effect of your eye contact with people who are threatening. It is often less provocative to use shorter periods of gaze than you might use normally. People who are very angry often use glaring eye contact and it is easy to get locked into unwittingly combative eye contact. Regular breaking of eye contact can help reduce this.

Think about relational levels also in situations like this. For example:

- Avoid standing over someone who is becoming angry

- Avoid sitting much lower down. This enhances the power of the angry person and also makes it more difficult for you to run away

- It may help if you 'mirror' or match the person's sitting or standing posture. As Linsley (2004) notes, this is a natural spontaneous action that can enhance communication if done well. But care must be taken not to exaggerate this activity or make it too obvious or silly as it may be misinterpreted as mocking the person. Generally speaking, most people do 'mirroring' naturally without thinking about it. Next time you are at a social gathering or party take time observing how people shape and alter their postures to match the person they are speaking to

- Use 'mood matching' if appropriate. Linsley (2004), for example, describes 'mood matching' as responding to the angry person with a 'similar level of energy', not in an aggressive sense, but as 'concern, involvement and interest'. This may avoid the risk of appearing uninterested by presenting a calm appearance – a usual response to aggression. Which option you choose will depend on your own assessment of the situation and the approach that seems the best to apply. If in doubt, then simply remain calm but focus on establishing through your comments that you are genuinely concerned and interested in the issues behind the person's anger or frustration

- Try to empathise without being patronising

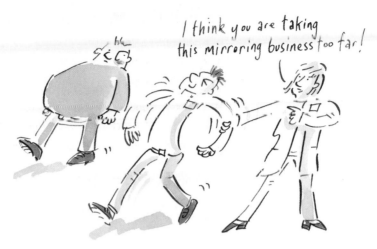

I think you are taking this mirroring business too far.

- Avoid making deals you can't keep
- Use your clarifying skills to communicate to the aggressor that you are trying to understand, but don't say: 'I understand', because you probably won't
- Try to avoid 'cornering' the person in any sense, either physically or psychologically.

The essential thing to remember in situations like this is to trust your instinct, gut feeling, or sixth sense. If that is telling you something is wrong, then respond to it rather than your intellect, which may be saying something different. You can spend all the time you need reflecting on your reaction later when you are safe (Bonham 2004, p. 15). Generally speaking, expert interventions are required when aggressiveness is at a high level or in violent situations. Here, more specialised approaches and training may be required (Beer *et al.* 2001, Stuart and Laraia 2001, Mason and Chandley 1999).

Key points | **Top tips**

When dealing with a patient who appears angry or frustrated:

- Assess the patient and the situation
- Assess your own personal safety
- Identify things that may be causing stress (stressors) and signs that a person is stressed
- Respond as early as possible – either removing yourself from the person if you feel threatened or engaging with the person

Top tips

- Maintain a large personal space
- Use a non-aggressive posture
- Use the option of either keeping calm or matching mood in terms of concern, involvement and interest (Linsley 2004) based on your own assessment of the situation
- Use person-centred verbal and non-verbal skills
- Speak clearly and calmly
- Provide key information that may be helpful to the person
- Avoid verbal struggles
- Maintain the patient's self-esteem and dignity through respectful, polite communication
- Establish what the patient considers to be their need
- Be goal oriented
- Invest time in being with the person
- Present several options or suggestions
- Remain honest and demonstrate genuineness and empathy
- Be assertive but not aggressive

Key points

- Health care environments can easily provoke conflict
- There are a number of interpersonal approaches that may at least help to partially diffuse or de-escalate such conflict
- Sometimes immediate actions are required to protect the safety of yourself and others
- In conflict situations learn to trust your instinct

Over to you

Read:

Linsley, P. (2004) 'Aggression'. In: *Nursing Knowledge and Practice: Foundations for Decision Making* (ed. Mallik, M. Hall, C. and Howard, D.), 2nd edition. Edinburgh: Balliere Tindall pp. 245–262.

Or:

Mason, T. and Chandley, M. (1999) *Managing Violence and Aggression: A Manual for Nurses and Health Care Workers*. Churchill Livingstone, Edinburgh.

●━ᴨ *Keywords*

Proactive
Taking the initiative in creating or controlling a situation

Dealing with an angry colleague

Dealing with an angry colleague can be more problematic to manage, in some ways, than the angry patient or relative. As you will have gathered from the examples above, often the tipping point or 'crisis' comes after a long period of 'simmering' about some issue. As mentioned, the ideal way to manage this kind of situation is to anticipate and therefore manage it a **proactive** way instead of reactively. That is, waiting for things to happen or 'get out of hand' before responding. Sometimes we, as nurses, are good at finding solutions for the patients and relatives we meet, but not quite so effective at managing issues that are 'in house'. The angry colleague is no different from the angry relative in the way that the communication can be dealt with as in the points indicated in 1–8 on p. 118. The difference is that you as a nurse may have to live close up with the consequences of your interaction, whether or not it is effective. Your colleague might be angry for a range of reasons:

1. Unjustifiably and/or chronically overworked (this is how they see it)
2. Under-appreciated. No-one acknowledges that they are overworked
3. Having to manage abuse from patients or relatives without any support
4. Having a grievance against a colleague
5. Upset or stressed by things outside of the work setting
6. Not being clear about their role in the work setting
7. Their role being eroded by others.

You will see that few of the above have an easily achieved or instant answer or resolution. Many of them you will be unable to address yourself. Therefore, realistically, your only role in this may be that of listener. Yet again, the person-centred approach can be helpful here. Adopting this strategy doesn't solve the problem but it can sometimes help you to defuse the anger, which after all is the immediate issue for Judy, the nurse in the following situation:

Paula: I'm really fed up with Pete. He's constantly trying to humiliate me in front of the rest of the staff. If he tries it again I'm going.
Judy: Going where?
Paula: Leaving. I'll get a job somewhere else.
Judy: So what exactly does he say? (*Clarifying*)
Paula: Last night I was sorting out the staff rota. He came in after I'd done it and started to mess about with what I'd arranged. He

said the night staff wouldn't be happy with it, right in front of that new manager.

Judy: That must have been a bit embarrassing. (*Attempting to be empathic*)

Paula: Well, I thought it was OK at first, I didn't mind too much. But then when I got home I started to think about things – he's always doing it.

Judy: Well, he likes to know what's going on, doesn't he? Perhaps he's just trying to keep people happy. (*Trying to be non-judgemental, looking at the other possibilities*)

Paula: Well, he's not keeping *me* happy. I'm going to tell him.

Judy: That's probably not a bad idea. (*Supportive*)

Paula: Do you think so?

Judy: At least he'll know how you feel. Then if he keeps doing it you'll know you were right. But give him a chance first? (*Being the 'grown up', trying out the options*)

In this example, you can see that no resolution is reached. There is, however, a step forward. Paula has been helped to see things a little more widely. She has also been supported by Judy as she attempts to progress the situation constructively. In the 'angry colleague' scenario, this is probably as much as you can hope to achieve 'briefly'. Unlike the first two situations regarding disgruntled patients and angry relatives, the difference here is that there is a high possibility of you becoming, or already being, part of the 'politics' of the situation, however much you try to keep your distance!

Key points Top tips

- Dealing with an angry colleague can be more problematic, to manage, in some ways, than the angry patient or relative

- There are a number of issues that may lead to a colleague becoming angry or frustrated: being overworked, under-appreciated, managing abuse from patients or relatives without support, having a grievance against a colleague, stressed by aspects of life outside the workplace, role confusion or role erosion

- Realistically, your only role in this may be that of listener, supporting the person in seeing 'all sides' in balanced and constructive steps toward finding a resolution.

Dealing with telephone complaints and reducing hosility

Managing complaints and hostility on the telephone presents another layer of difficulty to what can be already quite challenging for the nurse. The reason is that the essential information you can gain from seeing someone's body language as they express their frustration or anger is completely missing. It is important, therefore, that you make the most of what you've got and that is listening carefully to the language and **inflection**. The effective nurse will strive to 'hear' or interpret the needs of the caller and respond appropriately.

The less effective nurse, as in the following example, will fail to do this:

Nurse (*answers phone*): Hello Ward 4?
Caller: It's Alison again.
Nurse: Who? (*sounds impatient*)
Caller: I've just been speaking to a nurse there about my dad, Mr Wright. John Wright (*sounds agitated and frustrated*). I'm not happy with what I'm being told. I really want –
Nurse: (*Interrupts*) We haven't got a Mr Wright on here.
Caller: Yes, you have! Who am I speaking to? Are you in charge? I want to speak to the nurse in charge.
Nurse: Hold your horses! I'll just double check (*pauses and checks admission board*). Oh yeah, he's on the board.
Caller: Well, I'm worried about him. Is he all right? He was very poorly this morning. I want to know how he's doing. The other nurse hardly told me anything. I want to know how my father is. I want to –
Nurse: (*Interrupts*) You will have to ring back later. We're busy at the moment (*puts down the receiver*).

In the example above, we can see how the nurse fails in a very stark way to follow key strategies for the successful management of telephone complaints. These are as follows:

- Identify oneself *as well as* the clinical unit or area
- Be very polite
- Do not interrupt
- Listen carefully
- Demonstrate empathy
- Clarify key points by paraphrasing and summarising
- Strive to reduce hostility or conflict

Keywords

Inflection
Varying the tone or pitch of the voice

- Attempt to resolve queries or concerns
- Be the last to put down the receiver
- Follow-up any agreed actions.

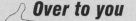

Over to you

Read:
Forsyth, P. (2000) *Telephone Skills*. London: Chartered Institute of Personnel and Development.

Key points　Top tips

- Managing complaints and hostility on the telephone presents another layer of difficulty to what can be already quite challenging for the nurse
- There are a number of key strategies for the successful management of telephone complaints, including identifying oneself, being polite, striving to reduce hostility or conflict and attempting to resolve queries or concerns

Breaking bad news

As with dealing with violent incidents, there are texts that deal in a specialised way with breaking bad news (e.g. Faulkner 1998) so here we will discuss some basic pointers only. First, it is important to appreciate that for the person in front of you what constitutes 'bad news' is a very personal thing. For example, bad news could be one or more of the following:

The person has . . .

. . . 6 months to live

. . . 10 years to live

. . . to take medication for a month

. . . to take medication for life

. . . to lose a limb

. . . to lose their hair

. . . to be admitted to hospital

. . . to stay in hospital for longer than anticipated.

əitəЯ*Reflective activity*

Think of some more examples from your own practice where you have had to break bad news.

How did you feel giving such news?

What kinds of responses did you witness?

What helps this process? What makes it difficult?

As discussed in Chapter 2, a person-centred approach will almost always help you when breaking bad news. That means you *attempt* to empathise, be accepting and be congruent (Bonham 2004). What these terms mean in the real life 'breaking bad news situation' is that you try to understand in some way how this person might be feeling about the bad news (or the news that is bad *to them*). You try to be accepting (or non-judgemental) of the person's response to the bad news (regardless of how you think you might feel in a similar situation). Finally, in terms of a person-centred approach, you try to be congruent (or honest or genuine) with the person who is dealing with the bad news in their own way. Here are some of the ways that a person hearing bad news could respond:

- They may get angry with the hospital staff, management, the NHS, you or your colleagues
- They may get angry with themselves. This can be shown externally by shouting or other demonstrations of temper, or internally as silence, **passivity** and withdrawal
- They may go into a form of shock, shaking, going pale, or feeling faint or weak. They may even surprise you with the speed at which they seem to be accepting of their bad news. This can be real, or it sometimes can be a form of denial. You will find some literature that argues the existence of grieving cycles (Worden 1991, cited in Walter 1999). A more contemporary view is that while for some people their grief seems to follow a traditional pattern, others seem to have their own way of doing it. Usually, people 'recover' in their own time. Sometimes if a person seems to be struggling with an unusually prolonged recovery, interventions by mental health professionals may be considered.

⚷ Keywords

Passivity
Being inactive, submissive or offering no opposition

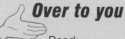

Over to you

Read:
Faulkner, A. (1998) *When the News is Bad. A guide for health professionals.*
Nelson Thornes, Cheltenham.

Key points   Top tips

- What constitutes 'bad news' is a very personal thing
- A person-centred approach will almost always help when breaking bad news
- A person hearing bad news could become angry at hospital staff, at themselves, or go into a form of shock
- Sometimes if a person seems to be struggling with an unusually prolonged recovery, interventions by mental health professionals may be considered

Communication with people who are anxious, stressed, depressed or confused

We will now consider the impact or effect of anxiety, stress, depression or confusion on communication and identify strategies to enhance interaction. It is worth noting that the four terms – anxiety, stress, depression and confusion – can be closely linked to each other in terms of a person's behaviour. That is, a person may suffer with all three at the same time. On the other hand it is important to remember that it is quite conceivable that a person could suffer from one or two of these without necessarily suffering from another. In other words a person might be depressed without being stressed or anxious, or anxious without being stressed or depressed, or confused and anxious and so on. You will see that it is important to try to work out which of these difficulties applies in each individual case.

In addition, it is important to bear in mind that some anxiety, stress and depression can be useful, necessary, appropriate and healthy. For example, in terms of anxiety a certain amount of adrenaline could serve to enhance performance, for example, in an examination or driving test. It can keep you focused if you have a deadline to work to (such as a course assignment). Again, stress is a part of all our lives, and can work to motivate us. Some people actively seek it out, for example, going on high thrill roller coaster rides or watching scary movies. Depression, where a person becomes low in mood can be thought of as a normal, healthy response following the loss of a loved one or end of a relationship. Most people would hesitate to start intervening in terms of 'treatments' or even considering that course of action in this instance. This would only be likely if such grieving did not resolve within a period of six to twelve months or it was interfering with the person's ability to 'carry on' with their normal functioning. Again, confusion can be a perfectly normal response to being overloaded with new information, subjected to an overwhelming series of events, or communication and miscommunication that requires interpretation.

Reflective activity

List the serious or significant losses that a person may experience across the lifespan.
How long is an appropriate time of grieving for each event?
What could be the signs of unhealthy or inappropriate grieving?

The first impact that anxiety, stress, depression or confusion can have is to affect a person's communication with others. The nurse has to see how communication is altered by carrying out a mini-assessment with the person.

Reflective activity

Consider how you feel when anxious, stressed, depressed or confused?
How does this manifest itself in your behaviour?
How does it affect your communication?

Feeling anxious or stressed

If a person is anxious or feeling stressed, they may seem distracted, fidgety, irritable and sensitive to noise. They may object to people getting too close to them (proximity) or touching them. They may also deny having a problem even when gently confronted:

Nurse: Simon, you look a bit on edge this morning.
Simon: No, I'm fine. No worries . . .

You can sometimes *hear* the incongruity in a person's voice if they are presenting a different mood or affect from the way that they are really feeling inside. Again, it can sometimes be helpful if the nurse tries to address this:

Nurse: Well, you say you are fine, but you don't look fine.
Simon: OK, I'm struggling today. I was better yesterday.

You can sometimes *see* the incongruity as well. Look out for uncharacteristic or unusual (for that person) signs: restlessness, fidgeting, blushing, flushing, going pale, sweating, shaking, excessive blinking, nail-biting, teeth-grinding (bruxism), hand-wringing. The person may be positioning themselves in what might be a hunched, defensive posture – arms tightly folded or legs wound around each other. They may be holding a hand across their face or mouth. It is often assumed, by the way, that these signals are always defensive. The effective nurse will always try to obtain *verbal confirmation* that what they are seeing is what that person is feeling:

Nurse: You actually look really wound up, Simon. Your knuckles are white and you're shaking.
Simon: Yes, OK! Just leave me alone will you? I've just about had enough!

Although Simon's response is blunt, the nurse has been *gently persistent* because she wants to know how he really is. Once this has been established, she will have some idea of how to start to help him. If she had not persisted, Simon would not have had the opportunity to express his true feelings.

Feeling 'low' or depressed

Depression can manifest itself in a number of ways. The person becomes 'absent' in an unusual way for them. That is, they may seem to be uncharacteristically disengaged from what is going on around them. This is to be expected as depression involves being negative about the self and others. Or the person may be absent in a very tangible way, that is, unable to function at their usual level in terms of many social and work settings. Features of this include: a tendency to lower the head or look downwards; slow, monotone speech; poor eye contact; slow movements; poor concentration, memory and decision-making; tearfulness; flat or blunted mood; irritability; excessive worrying; expressing that they have nothing to look forward to, feel worthless or want to die; changes in sleeping patterns (sleeping too much or too little); changes in eating patterns (again too much or too little); loss of libido or sex drive; loss of interest in things they would normally enjoy.

There is substantial evidence to suggest that many people who suffer from episodes of depression will recover *without* any professional intervention. Yet nurses without specific mental health training can help make a difference to people they meet who are suffering from depression by carefully adjusting the style of communication they adopt with them. This does not require in-depth knowledge and expertise – something that can be obtained from texts that are specifically aimed at mental health nurses (e.g. Stuart and Laraia 2001).

The main strategy here sounds simple – you just listen. If, however, you have experience of helping someone who is depressed, you will know that this needs some further elaboration.

'Just listening' can mean being more silent than you may be used to. People who are depressed may feel they have nothing to say to you, or anyone else. Your strategy then, is to maximise the opportunities for the person to speak to you, when they feel they can speak. And the 'speaking' may not be with words – it may be with just a gesture or a glance of the eyes. If you have spent time around the person 'just listening', you will have a greater chance of recognising this and responding to it, if and when it happens. Again, the person-centred model of communicating has a lot to offer us, in terms of our ability to help. If you try to empathise, try to be accepting (this can sometimes be difficult when what you will see is a person who will not respond 'normally' to your usual style of interacting) and be yourself, eventually if you are patient, consistent and gently persistent, the chances are that you will see some positive results from your work.

Communication with a confused person

The experience of confusion can be very distressing and the sensitive and effective nurse will always consider how best to communicate with such individuals. A common cause for confusion is dementia, which presents in various forms, most strikingly perhaps in Alzheimer's Disease. As Davies and Craig (1998) indicate, confusion is a 'state in which there is fluctuation in level of consciousness, with impairment of attention and memory'. Often, confusion results from difficulties with short-term memory and may be starkly apparent when an individual fails to identify or orient to time, place and person. Sometimes, individuals may struggle to recognise family members who they have known for a long time or even believe that relatives or partners who have died are still alive. But wherever confusion occurs, and independent of its cause and unique presentation, the following 'Top Tips' can act as a useful guideline in the process of interaction.

Key points **Top tips**

- Use simple, direct language that avoids 'flowery' or complicated speech
- Introduce tasks, information, thoughts or concepts ONE at a time
- Speak clearly and slowly
- Do not raise your voice as this could be misinterpreted as aggression and threat
- Do not used 'baby talk'
- Avoid sounding patronizing
- Be patient when the person is attempting or struggling to convey a message
- Do not ignore comments that do not seem to make sense but listen to 'content' and tone
- Tune in or heighten awareness of your own and the person's non-verbal communication
- Be aware that an inability to communicate can increase frustration and anger
- Avoid critical remarks or confronting any mistakes in terms of detail or accuracy the person makes
- Be aware of poor concentration and attention span
- Address the person by their name as this is polite, promotes **orientation** and a sense of belonging or identity
- Approach the person from the front, establish eye contact and do not attempt rapid, sudden or surprising communication
- Only use appropriate, not over-intrusive, touch
- In achieving tasks or giving information, chunk these down to small steps or amounts
- Use prompts and guide the person, making use of signs etc for orientation
- Promote retention of information by use of visual clues, symbols, photos, gestures, colour-coded objects or environmental areas etc

Keywords

Orientation
A person's adjustment to time, place and person

Key points Top tips

- The first impact that anxiety, stress, depression or confusion can have is to affect a person's communication with others
- The nurse has to see how communication is altered by carrying out a mini-assessment
- There are a number of verbal and non-verbal clues in assessing when a patient may be anxious, stressed, depressed or confused
- Listening and spending time with patients (even in silence) is essential

Communicating with people who do not speak English or where English is their second language

In clinical settings we can expect to meet a diverse range of people, including those who do not speak English or where English is their second language. We need to consider the communication needs of these people. Many readers of this book will have visited countries abroad for holidays, backpacking, and so on. Even if you haven't been in situations where English is not the first spoken language, it does not take much imagination to get a sense of how difficult it can be for people in heath care situations, especially when they do not speak English at all or where English is their second language. What may be commonplace phrases to us, such as 'I'll be with you in a minute', 'Hang in there', or 'It's all done and dusted' may be difficult to understand, even when people have a well-developed knowledge of English as a second language. Such individuals may struggle to comprehend some aspects of English usage and phrasing, not least health care jargon or the variations in expression that can exist in different regions of the UK.

Here is an approximate transcript of a conversation that took place in a gymnasium's sauna between a man (Speaker B) who enters and places a few drops of oil onto the coals and one of the authors (PB), who is marked as Speaker A:

Speaker A: That's a good idea. Is it eucalyptus?
Speaker B: Peppermint.
Speaker A: Excellent!

Long pause . . .

Speaker B: Do you know where liddle is?
Speaker A: Lidl?
Speaker B: Yes.
Speaker A: Do you know the big hospital? Well, it's the other side of that.
Speaker B: Do you understand deeveedee?
Speaker A: DVD?
Speaker B: Yes. The shop where I get DVD next to Lidl has closed. I get DVD for two nights. I am sorry. Do you know of anywhere in the city where I can get DVD?
Speaker A: No, not in the city. I can't think of anywhere apart from Blockbuster. That's a big shop north of the city.

This example is given here because it contains some features that demonstrate the difficulties that can occur in other settings, including health care, when communicating with patients who are not fluent English speakers.

As many of our cities and towns have diverse and multi-cultural populations, it is becoming increasingly rare to meet a nurse who has never been asked to manage situations where communication difficulties are primarily caused by differences in language.

In the conversation above, the English speaker is welcoming and supportive towards the other person. In the care setting you can do this easily – a genuine smile together with a warm voice tone (especially if the other person is sight impaired) is cross cultural and understood by everyone. It is worth trying words and phrases like 'hello', 'how are you?', 'thanks' with people who are not fluent in English as they may know a few key words. Combine these words together with an encouraging voice tone and some clear physical signals, and you may be surprised at what can be achieved. This 'sticking plaster' approach has severe limitations of course, and in health or clinical settings it is likely that you will need the services of an interpreter. In the meantime, returning to the scenario above, once the welcome signals have been sent and received, a tentative exploration then starts. The first question asked has nothing to do with the real issue, but it is a means to an end. Once Speaker B found that Speaker A knew where a Lidl store was then he knew it would be likely that he also knew the DVD rental shop nearby. Once that was established then there was a good chance that he would know where another DVD shop was. The communication, then, is a process of edging carefully forward, acknowledging where the communication breaks down because either the English speaker doesn't understand, or the non-English speaker doesn't know how to say it. Of course, health care encounters and the communication these require can be far more exacting than the example set out above, not least in terms of the serious nature of consultations and interventions and the likelihood that levels of anxiety and distress would figure prominently. As mentioned above, the latter can often be partially diffused by a welcoming affect and voice tone on the part of the professional.

Essentially then, the needs of non-English speaking people or those who speak English as a second language in health care settings are similar to ours. They require:

- information
- a friendly approach
- reassurance
- to be listened to.

Some of these needs can be met by clear non-verbal communication from nursing staff. Some can be met by sign boards, symbols and information leaflets that incorporate major non-English languages. But in many cases the needs of such individuals will only be fully met by use of a carefully chosen interpreter or within their own language community. Access to interpretation services is part of the national requirement for NHS Trusts meeting patient and public involvement guidance. This can be individual interpreters or, as has been taken up in some Trusts, through the adoption of 'Language Line' a 24-hour interpreting service linked to the bedside telephone/TV services.

The main ingredient in giving effective care in such difficult circumstances is a willingness to provide it, on the part of the care team. This willingness and a creative approach can overcome many obstacles when trying to help the non-English speaking patient or where confusion or misunderstanding occurs when communicating with individuals who may speak English as a second language yet require careful clarification of any unfamiliar phrases or expressions and their meaning.

Key points Top tips

- We need to consider the communication needs of people who do not speak English or where English is their second language
- Language barriers can be partially overcome by a welcoming affect, friendly tone of voice; use of common, simple words and clear non-verbal communication on the part of the professional; and sign boards, symbols and information leaflets that incorporate major non-English languages
- In many cases the needs of such individuals will only be fully met by use of a carefully chosen interpreter or within their own language community

RRRRR Rapid recap

Check your progress so far by working through each of the following questions:

1. What term can be applied to when frustration builds to crisis point?
2. What aspect of professional working can result in potential conflict with relatives making enquiries about a patient?
3. What term is used when referring to reducing anger or conflict?
4. What is the first thing you should do when answering a telephone call?
5. What mental health state might feature slow, flat or monotone speech?

If you have difficulty with more than one of the questions, read through the section again to refresh your understanding before moving on.

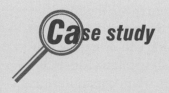

Case study

Read the following account of how a doctor informed a woman about the progress of her illness:

'He came in, and I'm in a quad room – four people – there's a few nurses around, a couple of cleaning ladies . . . Some people had company and he didn't even pull the curtains around my bed to tell me I had recurring cancer, and that I had a tumour the size of the hand, and that it was total removal if this (further treatment) was unsuccessful. Everybody was staring at me . . . I was just devastated . . . and he came back to me the next day and he said "I'm really sorry I did that", and I said, "Well, I know you must have a lot on your mind but the offence here is that you see me as a tumour, not as a person"' (Mathieson and Stam 1995, pp. 295–297).

● What approach should have been taken in breaking the bad news to this woman?
● How would you help or assist her in renegotiating her sense of identity?

References

Beer, D., Pereira, S. and Paton, C. (2001) *Psychiatric Intensive Care*. Greenwich Medical, Chatham.

Bonham, P. (2004) *Communicating as a Mental Health Carer*. Nelson Thornes, Cheltenham.

Davies, T. and Craig, T.K.J. (1998) *ABC of Mental Health*. BMJ Books, London.

Egan, G. (2002) *The Skilled Helper*, 7th edn. Brooks Cole, Pacific Grove, CA.

Faulkner, A. (1998) *When the News is Bad: A guide for health professionals*. Stanley Thornes, Cheltenham.

Forsyth, P. (2000) *Telephone Skills*. London: Chartered Institute of Personnel and Development.

Gillies, D. A. (1994) *Nursing Management. A systems approach*, 3rd edn. W.B. Saunders, Philadelphia.

Harrison, A. and Hart, C. (eds) (2006) *Mental Health Care for Nurses: Applying mental health skills in the general hospital.* Blackwell Publishing, Oxford.

Linsley, P. (2004) 'Aggression'. In: *Nursing Knowledge and Practice: Foundations for decision making*, 2nd edn, (eds Mallik, M., Hall, C. and Howard, D.) Edinburgh: Balliere Tindall. pp. 245–262.

Marelli, T. M. (1997) *The Nurse Manager's Survival Guide*, 2nd edn. Mosby, St Louis, MD.

Mason, T. and Chandley, M. (1999) *Managing Violence and Aggression: A manual for nurses and health care workers.* Churchill Livingstone, Edinburgh.

Mathieson, C.M. and Stam, H.J. (1995) Re-negotiating identity: Cancer narratives. *Sociology of Health and Illness*, **17**(3): 295–297.

Stuart, G. and Laraia, M. (2001) *Principles and Practice of Psychiatric Nursing.* Mosby, St Louis, YMO.

Walter, T. (1999) *On Bereavement: The culture of grief.* Open University Press, Buckingham.

6 ▶ Brief, Ordinary and Effective (BOE): A new model for health care communication

Learning outcomes

By the end of this chapter you should be able to:

- Appreciate the value of brief, ordinary communication

- Acknowledge the need for effective, evidence-based communication

- Look for opportunities in clinical settings to enhance the communication experience of patients.

Brief communication

There is nowadays a more or less universal recognition that communication skills are a key element of any contemporary clinician's skill repertoire and are essential to their competence, yet a major issue facing health care professionals is that of finding time for communication with clients. Lack of time is a key factor in clinical life, something that some studies show rules out the practice of evidence-based medicine (McColl *et al.* 1998; Tomlin *et al.* 1999; Young and Ward 2001). These days, health practitioners are increasingly task driven, burdened with administration and concerned to boost their 'people processing'. This is so much the case that communication can be perceived as something that slows down or can 'get in the way' of health care encounters, whether it is preparing nursing home residents for bed, administering injections or weighing infants. From the clients' point of view such a businesslike approach that avoids communication is often most unsatisfactory and can lead to a sense of alienation and complaints that care is superficial, oppressive, humiliating or inhumane. Indeed, where clients are confused or require reassurance lack of communication might even lead to violence.

At present a good deal of health care training is driven by an implicit model that views counselling as the ideal to which practitioners should aspire. Yet the busy nature of many clinical settings makes it difficult to achieve this more extended form of communication based around counselling notions of therapeutic relationships, deepening empathy and mutual storytelling. As a result, clinicians have viewed communication as something that takes up a lot of time and therefore overlooked the opportunities of maximising targeted rather than open-ended communication – something that

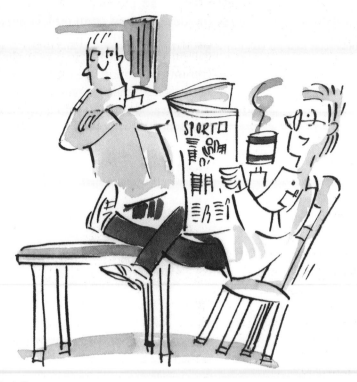

Time to talk.

fits the organisational constraints and demands of modern health care where clinicians are driven ever more firmly towards brevity.

In order to achieve rapid, effective and emotionally supportive communications, practitioners need a reality-driven conception of communicative practice that moves away from time-greedy communication by extracting the best elements from counselling models and applying them to the 'time sensitive' situation of busy health care settings.

To make sense of this and develop some recommendations for practice we will introduce the Brief, Ordinary and Effective (BOE) model of communication. While the kinds of evidence available to support these components of therapeutic communication will necessarily be of a different category than laboratory science, it leads us to consider a new **paradigm** for health care communication that moves away from counselling in promoting briefer yet satisfying forms of interaction. This paradigm or model is not to be followed religiously, in a narrow fashion like a **protocol** – telling you what to do – or something you can tick boxes for, but is intended as a map of key aspects of communication that are considered valuable and around which you can develop your existing skills based on past experience. The aim is to stimulate new learning and practice, and

Keywords

Paradigm
An example or pattern

Protocol
A set of rules or procedure

the development of an ethical personality that seeks to be a good practitioner to the benefit of patients and clients. In so doing, we will outline strategies in accomplishing brief, ordinary and effective communication in the often demanding environments of health care settings and make suggestions as to how this communication can be incorporated into the education and training of future health professionals.

> **Key points** Top tips
>
> - Lack of time is a key factor in clinical life
> - Communication can be perceived as something that can 'get in the way' of health care encounters
> - Time-greedy counselling is often the ideal to which practitioners aspire
> - Modern health care requires a new model that promotes brief, ordinary and effective communication

Brief communication can be powerful

Brief communication is that which provides succinct, essential information and is of short duration, or as Ben Jonson writes: 'The brief style is that which expresseth much in little.' This communication can be spoken, written, non-verbal or involve the use of images or symbols. Nearly a quarter of a century ago Alvin Toffler (1980) envisioned a future characterised by what he called 'blip culture' where 'we are increasingly exposed to short . . . blips of information – adverts, commands, theories, shreds of news . . .' (p. 182). In the same way, a great many health care encounters take place in short 'blips' often of 5 minutes or less across a range of sites and involve a vast number of practitioners. From acute admissions wards to nursing homes, from scanner suites to complementary practitioners, NHS walk-in centres to plastic surgeons, the public encounter a variety of fragments of health care communication. As we have outlined earlier, what is needed is a comprehensive model of how all these brief encounters can be part of the therapeutic environment.

This will be a practical chapter and we will aim to distil from our reference to existing literature throughout this book and our own research, a set of guidelines for health care encounters of five minutes or less, and emphasise how even momentary communications can convey support, warmth and a sense of inclusion. For example, it should be possible to communicate meaningfully even in passing in a corridor or through a ward and provide comfort and support 'on the hoof'. The skill element in communication might be more to do with strategies for identifying and responding to opportunities for interaction – therefore, successful health care communicators may be those who adapt to task-dominated environments and utilise even momentary time slots to good effect Brown *et al.* (2006). This backcloth of successive momentary engagement and warmth could create a positive realm for recovery. We might think of this as a rich, pervasive atmosphere that patients can benefit from. As Argyle (1994) indicates, liking other people is signalled by smiling, gaze, proximity, touch, open posture and higher pitch of voice, all of which are not 'time-greedy' and can be achieved without what we might call 'time-anxiety'.

We know, from the discussion in Chapter 2, that brief forms of communication such as eye contact, nodding, smiling, friendly or humorous small-talk (phatic communication), touch, facial, hand or body gestures are vital to establishing and sustaining rapport with other people. These can be seen as an ordinary yet key aspect of creating, sustaining and terminating therapeutic relationships with patients/clients. This **synchronous communication** can be done while carrying out other tasks and duties.

○━┓ *Keywords*

Synchronous communication

Communication which occurs at the same time as another activity, or while completing another task

Top tips

- Make a point of acknowledging *all* the patients in your clinical setting when you come on duty through eye contact, a nod, smile or the exchange of a few words
- Seize all opportunities to communicate warmth and acceptance while carrying out tasks with patients

Box 6.1: Brief, Ordinary, Effective (BOE) – Summary of a new model for communication in health care

Given the demands on contemporary health care professionals, and the limited time to carry out interventions, it is crucial that optimal brief encounters or interactions take place that are ordinary yet effective. The rationale for BOE lies in an evidence base that suggests:

1. **B**rief forms of communication such as eye contact, nodding, smiling, friendly or humorous small-talk or phatic communication, touch, facial, hand or body gestures are vital to establishing and sustaining rapport with other people.

2. **O**rdinary forms of communication create, sustain and terminate therapeutic relationships with patients/clients; reduce misunderstanding caused by expert language or jargon; and promote greater equality in interactions.

3. **E**ffective forms of communication bring about desirable outcomes in terms of patient satisfaction, elicit or provide accurate information or advice, and promote constructive interactions.

By focusing on such brief, ordinary and effective forms of communication practitioners working in health settings may bring about desirable outcomes in terms of patient satisfaction, gain or provide accurate information or advice, and promote constructive interactions within a time-constraining culture.

The impetus for considering brevity as a strategy in health care communication comes from several sources. First, our observations of communication in health care have suggested a curious contradiction. In clinical sites the brief kinds of jolly, supportive or encouraging communication that we use in everyday life, for example with friends and family, often disappears. In other words professionals seem to adopt formal, 'neutral' expressions in preference to ordinary and emotionally generous remarks or gestures. Sometimes, whereas the briefest of conversations with a friend can leave one with a good and lasting feeling of self-worth, the kinds of neglectful or unemotional exchanges in clinical sites can leave clients or patients feeling very isolated and ignored. The strengths of brief, kind, ordinary and friendly exchanges appear overlooked in health care.

Traditionally, health communication in nursing education has focused on teaching counselling skills (associated with professionalism and expertise) or processing skills (associated with business and economic efficiency). But the simpler, briefer interactions, such as a genuine rather than scripted smile, are taken for granted. It is assumed that such basic, valuable and powerful human interactions occur naturally and do not require monitoring or evaluation; that these kinds of exchanges do not deserve special attention.

This may not be the case and busy health professionals need to strive and consider how to make the best use of the few minutes, or even seconds, of consultation time available to them. After all, they are increasingly called upon to demonstrate the effectiveness not only of specific interventions but of their role as a whole. Given this perspective, it is perhaps the right time in the evolving world of health care that places such emphasis on technical expertise, to pay closer attention to the kinds of communication that support the notion of society, belonging, and create a sense of hope. Practitioners are often perfectly capable of making friends and family members feel good from a very brief interaction. Yet this kind of communication does not always get used in professional contexts.

There are many different sources of information in the literature about how mood and emotion are related to communication. There are research studies indicating the importance of communicative features such as greetings or compliments. There is also a strand of scholarship called speech act theory which stresses the fact that words *do* things. Communicating is an action that can have real physical, psychological and social consequences, as we suggested in Chapter 1. In this sense what we say or write, signal by image or symbol, *performs* rather than merely describes – *it acts* – it does things. For example, the 'small talk' or phatic communication that we referred to in Chapter 2 does things at a social level – it creates emotional togetherness, warmth and belonging.

The more traditional focus on specialist, time-greedy forms of communication in terms of counselling are implicitly content and problem-focused. A new emphasis on form over content in brief communication will afford a sustaining backdrop of warm, human interaction that:

- ensures a more affirmative interpersonal environment
- provides the basis for more 'time-greedy' and specialist communication such as counselling.

In a technology-driven health care environment, with its emphasis on processing patients, it is encouraging to note that health care practitioners are seeing the gap that has opened up in terms of providing an emotionally supportive and communicative environment. Bolton (2001) documents how experienced nurses manage the emotional content of their working lives. There is a sense even among these nurses that they could or should do more:

> *I went home the other night thinking I could have been kinder to Mr So and So. After all he is really worried about his wife and it's not up to him to know what sort of day it had been. But it was all I could do to present him with the facts in a calm, empty sort of way. I was on the brink of bawling myself, we'd had eight miscarriages and two deaths and I was worn out with it all. But I feel really sorry now that he didn't get what he should have got. I'm sure he'll be back. I suspect his wife is in for a run, so I'll try to make it up another time.*
>
> (Senior Staff Nurse). (Bolton 2001, p. 92)

There is evidence that patients want more and deeper connections with nurses (Shattell 2002, 2004). Patients experience the hospital environment as disconnecting and actively seek ways to connect with nurses. Their dependence on nursing staff, as well as perceived powerlessness in relation to that of the nurse, creates a situation where patients believe they have 'actively' to find ways to solicit the nursing care they need.

Demonstrating a willingness simply to be briefly, yet in a confirmatory way, in the presence of patients or service users may be beneficial. Making oneself visible to patients, their carers or relatives, and colleagues can provide reassurance and comfort without necessarily demanding further input in terms of time. It may be quite the opposite, where the inability to see health practitioners due to architectural limitations or their preference to remain 'hidden' in offices or stations provokes more use of bed-side buzzers, simply to assuage anxieties exacerbated by feelings of invisibility or isolation. Again, staff may feel inherently more supported and 'backed up' if their colleagues are visible to them, especially in challenging health environments.

Key points

- Brief encounters dominate health care delivery
- Practitioners need to adapt to task-dominated environments and utilise even momentary time slots to good effect
- Momentary and synchronous communication can convey support, warmth and a sense of inclusion
- A fundamental aspect of care is providing an emotionally supportive and communicative environment

The value of ordinariness

The quality of ordinariness that is so valued in human communication involves both verbal and non-verbal aspects. For example, just as much as people appear to enjoy casual conversational exchanges, it can also be rewarding to be in the company of another person who is being, behaving or has an ordinary or non-formal persona – perhaps accepting and unwrapping a sweet, smelling the flowers that have been brought in for a patient or drinking tea with them. Such activity is hardly 'time-greedy' – lasting seconds or at most (in the case of a cup of tea) a few minutes. Yet this presentation of the self can be helpful, for example, as part of a 'relationship-building skills repertoire' (Bonham 2004). On an intense, serious or alienating ward environment, such ordinariness can promote a certain homeliness and reassurance to patients. Be prepared to defend a level of ordinariness in your clinical settings, especially if subjected to narrow-minded complaints that this is not 'professional' or 'efficient'.

As we noted in Chapter 2, ordinary talk and 'ordinariness' in our presentation of ourselves presents no threat and encourages our relationships with patients and clients, promoting in them feelings of equality and belonging, and facilitating 'emotional agreement'. As Burnard (2003) noted, when talking about mental health nurses, '[they] may be remembered as much for their friendliness and ordinariness as for their counselling skills. Ordinary chat might be as important as therapeutic conversation' (p. 682). As Bonham (2004) indicates, this 'ordinariness' and 'real' approach can extend to how we offer suggestions for solving particular problems or probe and examine what people say to us, bringing matters 'down to earth', rather than speaking with a neutralised, professional style. Equally, everyday, ordinary speech patterns can offer a great deal of information about what really matters to people. For example, in the following statement, as Fritz Perls would have it, 'Everything before the *but* is bullshit' (McLeod 2003, p.162):

'My named nurse is very nice and she means well *but* I don't think she really understands where I'm coming from.'

Reflective activity

Consider the ways you use ordinary conversation in a purposeful way while caring for patients.

What topics do you tend to focus on when making 'small talk'?

Top tips

- Be yourself. Be ordinary. Ordinary *is* extraordinary
- It is exhausting to act or be something you are not
- Being genuine will help you get in touch with yourself and stay in touch with others

When thinking about ordinariness, and what this is in terms of communication, it is possible to gain some insight from the study of people gaining competence at a second language. Here it is widely acknowledged that there is far more to developing competence with a new or second language than merely learning the words and grammar. It is about achieving a style that does justice to the practical, everyday, small talk in the culture in question. That is, the work the language does to facilitate social interaction, agreeable experience, positive mood and even a sense of politeness amongst the speakers. In most contexts, the closer the interaction comes to what is taken to be 'ordinary conversation' in that culture then the more readily such desirable outcomes can be facilitated. Lakoff (1989, pp. 102–103), for instance, states that ordinary conversation functions as a template or frame for other forms of interaction 'which we experience in terms of their similarities to and differences from ordinary conversation and feel more or less comfortable with to the degree that they conform to our ordinary-conversation-based expectations'.

In considering second language learning, Richards (1990, p. 74) claims that 'the ability to produce this kind of casual conversational language as well as to produce language appropriate for more formal encounters is an essential skill for second language learners'. It may be beneficial for staff and clients in health care if they can be more aware of the relative merits of casual and formal communication, ensuring that the warmer, more informal conversation and interaction does not get squeezed out. Implementing what they know about how to hold a conversation outside the clinical context may well improve practitioners' work with clients.

Key points

Ordinariness:

- is valued in human communication
- presents no threat and encourages our relationships with patients and clients, promoting in them feelings of equality and belonging, and facilitating 'emotional agreement'
- can bring matters 'down to earth
- is about achieving a style that does justice to the practical, everyday, small talk in the culture in question

Effective or evidence-based communication

In essence, an evidence-based focus on communication can break the logjam of traditional counselling approaches in health care training that are more suited to mental health contexts. It promotes quick, general and practical communication along an axis of skilled ordinariness.

Throughout this book it has been our aim to offer some indication of the evidence base that supports the value of brief, ordinary and effective forms of communication, and to confirm the powerful and potentially transforming nature of these in health care practice.

Box 6.2: BOE core skills

1. Making oneself approachable and available to service users, their carers or relatives, colleagues, and partners from other statutory and non-statutory services

2. Demonstrating basic interpersonal skills in terms of appropriate eye contact, posture, proximity, relaxed manner, touch

3. Welcoming and initiating friendly and appropriate conversation

4. Conducting and sustaining polite, balanced, shared conversation with appropriate turn-taking and use of non-verbal and verbal prompts, i.e. head nods and hand gestures; phrases such as: 'go on', 'I see', 'okay'; and expressions such as 'uh-huh'

5. Ending or closing conversation in a mutually satisfying and respectful manner

6. Creating and sustaining rapport with others through active listening, attending, reflecting feelings, warmth, empathy, genuineness, being non-judgmental and accepting

7. Frequently acknowledging others by using brief, positive greetings, ordinary/ everyday conversation, or by engaging non-verbally, for example through eye contact, smiling and nodding

8. Using empowering language that encourages self-determination and decision-making of others

9. Using non-stigmatising language – avoiding the use of labels or descriptions that isolate, belittle or are abusive to others

10. Using dignified or self-respecting language

11. Negotiating care with service users in the spirit of concordance (reaching agreement)

12. Using simple activities to promote relationships with service users, such as bed- making, helping with meals, making a drink, washing, or mobilising, etc.

13. Demonstrating appropriate use of silence, for example in facilitating reflection, expression of feelings, conveying empathy; to encourage response to open questions; as an opportunity to observe or convey interest

14. Demonstrating appropriate use of humour to create an open, responsive social atmosphere; relax others and reduce stress; reach out to and engage others; increase interaction; and boost morale

15. Demonstrating a willingness simply to be in the presence of service users

16. Giving feedback to others that is constructive and facilitates positive change

17. Receiving and giving appropriate consideration to feedback from service users, carers, relatives and colleagues

18. Accurately interpreting and confirming (under supervision) non-verbal communication from service users, carers, relatives, and colleagues

19. Using appropriate open or closed questioning, being aware that asking too many questions may be stressful

20. Responding to questions in an honest and clear manner

21. Clarifying or checking out the meaning of what people say by careful use of questioning, summarising and paraphrasing. This is especially important when dealing with complex issues

22. Demonstrating sensitivity to the communication needs of people when English is their second language
23. Brief, time-limited counselling applied to specific service user situations (under supervision)
24. Communicating appropriately with individuals who have visual, hearing, speech or cognitive disabilities.
25. Identifying anxiety, depression and confusion and how these may affect communication ability
26. Identifying anger and frustration and using verbal and non-verbal de-escalation techniques
27. Providing sensitive, emotional support to colleagues and team members
28. Providing accurate advice, instruction, information and professional opinion to service users, carers, relatives and colleagues; and when necessary to groups of colleagues or service users/carers/relatives
29. Maintaining confidentiality in both spoken and written communication
30. Answering telephone enquiries in an appropriate manner: identifying oneself, being polite, striving to reduce hostility or conflict, resolving queries or concerns
31. Keeping brief, factual and accurate care records

Let us summarise now the key ingredients or core skills of the BOE Model for Health Communication that arise from the discussions in this and previous chapters. We contend that most of these components have limited time impact and can be achieved on a regular basis, unlike specialist counselling. In other words, they can be delivered in all health settings regardless of how busy they are.

For the BOE model to become established within health settings, a response is required by individual practitioners, education providers, and the health care trusts or institutions. By way of conclusion, let us indicate these briefly in turn:

- Individual practitioners need to develop and apply the skills of brief and ordinary interaction, seeking out further evidence to support communication approaches or strategies tailored to specific care environments and that work in the best interests of patients and clients
- Education providers need to incorporate teaching on brief and ordinary communication in the training of health practitioners, developing an evidence-based curriculum that utilises the latest advances in language and communication research and fully considers the reality of time-constraints in health care practice
- Health care trusts and services need to prioritise and promote the development of communication with an explicit focus on

creating a culture that values this activity as much as 'processes' and 'tasks' and rewards excellence and leadership in this field. In addition, such institutions should ensure that bureaucratic and other organisational activities and demands on health practitioners are kept 'lean and mean' to afford maximum opportunity for communication with patients. This 'space' for communicating with patients should be reviewed and audited.

Ensuring that health care professionals can work with patients and clients so as to sensitively take account of differences in background, values and lifestyle, and to respect human rights and promote human dignity, is of major importance in achieving policy objectives which set the patient at the heart of care. In the long term, effective communication is best served by awareness rather than protocols or 'do-lists'. The ability to use critical skills and adopt theoretical constructs while keeping in mind the humanitarian values of health care may ultimately serve professionals and clients better than an approach that ticks all the boxes.

Key points

- Skilled ordinariness incorporates quick, general and practical communication
- Practitioners should use brief, ordinary and effective forms of communication
- Individual practitioners, education providers and health care organisations need to work together to advance successful communication with patients

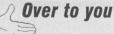 **Over to you**

Read:

Shattell. M. (2004) Nurse–patient interaction: a review of the literature, *Journal of Clinical Nursing*, **13**, 714–722.

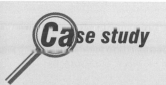 **Case study**

The following examples of conversation take place between a nurse and patient:

Nurse:	Morning, Sally. Get any sleep?
Sally:	Not really.
Nurse:	Try not to worry too much about that. You'll catch up when you're ready. Even a couple of hours is better than nothing. It's understandable that your sleep is disturbed, given what's happened, and that you're in a strange environment. How about some breakfast?
Sally:	I'll give it a miss. I don't usually bother at home.

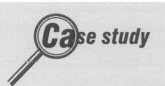
Case study

Nurse: I'll bring you a cup of tea in a while. See how you go.
Nurse: Hi, Sally. How about going for a walk with me for 20 minutes?
Sally: No, I'm all right.
Nurse: There's a patient's meeting in about an hour. You'd be very welcome. You don't have to say anything.
Sally: No, I'm OK, thanks. Meetings aren't my cup of tea.
Nurse: Some other time perhaps. They are once a week in the day room. If you want anything from the shop, let me know and we could walk down together. You must be sick of looking at these walls.
Sally: Yes, but I'd rather be here than in that flat.
Nurse: What was so bad about the flat?
Sally: It was starting to feel like a prison.
Nurse: How do you mean – a prison?

(Bonham 2004, pp. 87–88)

- How does the nurse develop a brief, meaningful strategy of ordinariness?
- What evidence is there in the interaction that this is a successful approach to adopt?

RRRRRRapid recap

Check your progress so far by working through each of the following questions.

1. What does the acronym BOE stand for?
2. Which specialist form of communication has dominated approaches to communication in health care?
3. Which term can be used to describe a society where brief forms of communication occur?
4. Which term is applied to communication that occurs at the same time as another activity, or while completing another task?
5. Which two key qualities did Burnard (2003) place above the ability to provide counselling?

If you have difficulty with more than one of the questions, read through the section again to refresh your understanding.

References

Argyle, M. (1994) *The Psychology of Interpersonal Behaviour*. Penguin, London.

Bolton, S.C. (2001) Changing faces: Nurses as emotional jugglers. *Sociology of Health and Illness*, **23**(1), 85–100.

Bonham, P. (2004) *Communicating as a Mental Health Carer*. Nelson Thornes, Cheltenham.

Brown, B., Crawford, P. and Carter, R. (2006) *Evidence-based Health Communication*. Open University Press: Maidenhead.

Burnard, P. (2003) Ordinary chat and therapeutic conversation: Phatic communication and mental health nursing. *Journal of Psychiatric and Mental Health Nursing*, **10**, 678–682.

Lakoff, R.T. (1989) The limits of politeness: Therapeutic and courtroom discourse. *Multilingua*, **8**, 101–129.

McColl, A., Smith, H., White, P. and Field, J. (1998) General practitioners' perceptions of the route to evidence based medicine: a questionnaire survey. *British Medical Journal*, **316**, 361–365.

McLeod, J. (2003) *An Introduction to Counselling*, 3rd edn. Open University Press: Buckingham.

Richards, J.C. (1990) *The Language Teaching Matrix*. Cambridge University Press, Cambridge.

Shattell, M. (2002) Eventually it'll be over: the dialectic between confinement and freedom in the phenomenal world of the hospitalized patient. In: *Listening to Patients: A phenomenological approach to nursing research and practice* (eds Thomas S. and Pollio H.) New York: Springer, pp. 214–236.

Shattell, M. (2004) Nurse–patient interaction: A review of the literature. *Journal of Clinical Nursing*, **13**, 714–722

Toffler, A. (1980) *The Third Wave*. William Morrow & Co, New York.

Tomlin, Z., Humphrey, C. and Rogers S. (1999) General practitioners' perceptions of effective health care. *British Medical Journal*, **318**, 1532–1535.

Young J.M. and Ward J.E. (2001) Evidence-based medicine in general practice: Beliefs and barriers among Australian GPs. *Journal of Evaluation in Clinical Practice*, **7**(2), 201–210.

Appendix

Rapid Recap – answers

Chapter 1

1. **What are the two key, basic models of communication?**
1. The two key, basic models of communication are:
   a. transmission
   b. transaction.

2. **Which area of the brain is involved in the production of speech?**
2. The area of the brain involved in the production of speech is Broca's area.

3. **What term is sometimes applied to the organisation and design of society?**
3. The term that is sometimes applied to the organisation and design of society according to particular viewpoints, norms or rules is social construction.

4. **What special term can be used in reference to activities such as praising, warning, promising or apologising?**
4. The special term that can be used in reference to activities such as praising, warning, promising, or apologising is speech acts.

5. **What do we call the patronising child-like speech used with older adults considered frail?**
5. We call the patronising, child-like speech used with older adults considered frail – secondary baby talk.

Chapter 2

1. **What can a higher pitch of voice convey?**
1. A higher pitch of voice conveys interest and engagement.

2. **What promotes attraction or likeability; indicates attentive listening and encourages disclosure?**
2. Smiling promotes attraction or likeability; indicates attentive listening and encourages disclosure.

3. **What is the formal term for 'chit chat' or 'small talk'?**
3. Phatic conversation or communication is the formal term for 'chit chat' or 'small talk'.

4. **What do you call the exchange, return or reciprocation of eye contact?**
4. The exchange, return or reciprocation of eye contact is called mutual gaze.

5. **What does the acronym SOLER stand for?**
5. The acronym SOLER stands for facing people SQUARELY, maintaining an OPEN shape to the body, LEANING forward slightly, using appropriate EYE CONTACT, RELAXING.

Chapter 3

1. **What are Peplau's six nursing roles?**
1. Peplau's six nursing roles are Counsellor, Leader, Surrogate, Stranger, Resource, Teacher.

2. What are the six categories of Heron's (1990) intervention analysis?

2. The six categories of Heron's (1990) intervention analysis are:

   a. Prescriptive

   b. Informative

   c. Confronting

   d. Cathartic

   e. Catalytic

   f. Supportive.

3. Which approach takes all aspects of a person into account not just the illness?

3. The holistic approach takes all aspects of a person into account not just the illness.

4. What is the word for when we are thinking in the same way as we behave?

4. The word for when we are thinking the same as we behave is congruent.

5. What are the two key activities related to clarifying?

5. The two key activities related to clarifying are:

   a. paraphrasing

   b. summarising.

Chapter 4

1. What word refers to reaching a harmonious agreement?

1. The word that refers to reaching a harmonious agreement is concordance.

2. What is another word for a label or mark that is associated with disgrace or undermines a person's character or identity?

2. The word 'stigma' is another word for a label or mark that is associated with disgrace or undermines a person's character or identity.

3. Berg (1996) refers to health care records as a 'semi-public' what?

3. Berg (1996) refers to health care records as a 'semi-public' memory.

4. Which professional body requires that nurses provide 'relevant information about the condition of the patient or client at any given time and the measures you have taken to respond to their needs'?

4. The Nursing and Midwifery Council is the professional body that requires nurses to provide 'relevant information about the condition of the patient or client at any given time and the measures you have taken to respond to their needs'.

5. Which three Acts of Parliament permit access by patients to all manual health records whenever made, subject to specified exceptions?

5. The THREE Acts of Parliament that permit access by patients to all manual health records whenever made, subject to specified exceptions are: Access to Health Records Act (1990), Data Protection Act (1998) and Human Rights Act (2000).

Chapter 5

1. What term can be applied to when frustration builds to crisis point?

1. The term can be applied to when frustration builds to crisis point is 'flashpoint'.

2. What aspect of professional working can result in potential conflict with relatives making enquiries about a patient?

2. Maintaining confidentiality is the aspect of professional working that can result in potential conflict with relatives making enquiries about a patient.

3. What term is used when referring to reducing anger or conflict?

3. De-escalation is the term that is used when referring to reducing anger or conflict.

4. What is the first thing you should do when answering a telephone call?

4. The first thing that you should do when answering a telephone call is identify yourself.

5. What mental health state might feature slow, flat or monotone speech?

5. Depression is the mental health state that might feature slow, flat or monotone speech.

Chapter 6

1. **What does the acronym BOE stand for?**

1. The acronym BOE stands for Brief, Ordinary, Effective.

2. **Which specialist form of communication has dominated approaches to communication in health care?**

2. Counselling is the specialist form of communication that has dominated approaches to communication in health care.

3. **Which term can be used to describe a society where brief forms of communication occur?**

3. The term that can be used to describe a society where brief forms of communication occur is blip culture.

4. **Which term is applied to communication that occurs at the same time as another activity, or while completing another task?**

4. Synchronous communication is the term that is applied to communication that occurs at the same time as another activity, or while completing another task.

5. **Which two qualities did Burnard (2003) place above the ability to provide counselling?**

5. The two key qualities Burnard (2003) placed above the ability to provide counselling are:

   a. friendliness

   b. ordinariness.

Index

Page reference in italics indicate figures or tables